INSTRUCTOR'S

to Accompa

Delmar's

Comprehensive Medical Terminology

A COMPETENCY-BASED APPROACH

Betty Davis Jones

Delmar Publishers

an International Thomson Publishing company ITP®

Albany • Bonn • Boston • Cincinnati • Detroit • London • Madrid
Melbourne • Mexico City • New York • Pacific Grove • Paris • San Francisco
Singapore • Tokyo • Toronto • Washington

By Delmar Publishers

an International Thomson Publishing Company, Inc.

The ITP logo is a trademark under license.

Printed in the United States of America

For more information, contact:

Delmar Publishers
3 Columbia Circle, Box 15015
Albany, New York 12212-5015

International Thomson Publishing Europe
Berkshire House
168-173 High Holborn
London, WC1V7AA
United Kingdom

Nelson ITP, Australia
102 Dodds Street
South Melbourne,
Victoria, 3205 Australia

Nelson Canada
1120 Birchmont Road
Scarborough, Ontario
M1K 5G4, Canada

International Thomson Publishing France
Tour Maine-Montparnasse
33 Avenue du Maine
75755 Paris Cedex 15, France

International Thomson Editores
Seneca 53
Colonia Polanco
11560 Mexico D. F. Mexico

International Thomson Publishing GmbH
Königswinterer Strasße 418
53227 Bonn
Germany

International Thomson Publishing Asia
60 Albert Street
#15-01 Albert Complex
Singapore 189969

International Thomson Publishing Japan
Hirakawa-cho Kyowa Building, 3F
2-2-1 Hirakawa-cho, Chiyoda-ku,
Tokyo 102, Japan

ITE Spain/ Paraninfo
Calle Magallanes, 25
28015-Madrid, Espana

ISBN 0-7668-0495-X

Library of Congress Catalog Number: 98-39257

Contents

Chapter Exams / 61

Answer Keys to Chapter Review Sheets / 167

Answer Keys to Chapter Exams / 197

References / 205

Practice Software Tutorial / 209

How to Use the Manual

COURSE SYLLABUS

The *Instructor's Manual for Comprehensive Medical Terminology* provides a two-semester course syllabus format as a guide in setting up the course. The instructor will note that the syllabus is based on a course that meets 3 days a week (1 hour each day) for 16 weeks in the semester, for a total of 48 contact hours.

The syllabus format included in this manual allows for the first day of class to cover course expectations, etc. Additionally, the assignments are listed by number of days devoted to the topic, with the number of hours devoted to the topic being noted also. Exam days are provided in the syllabus. The instructor can adjust the schedule and the number of exams as desired, to suit his/her needs for the course.

SUGGESTED CLASSROOM ACTIVITIES

The instructor will also find numerous suggested classroom activities to enhance the learning and to offer alternate teaching methods. These activities are explained in detail and samples are provided where appropriate.

CHAPTER REVIEW SHEETS

Chapter Review Sheets are provided for each chapter in the textbook, with the number of review sheets ranging from 2-6. These review sheets concentrate on word elements and stimulate the student to learn word elements in two ways: from definition to word element, and from word element to definition. This should reinforce the student's comprehension of the medical terms. Answers for all chapter review sheets are included at the end of the *Instructor's Manual.*

CHAPTER EXAMS

Each chapter in the text has an accompanying 50 question chapter exam that concentrates on the content of the chapter. Chapters 5-23 (that concentrate on body systems and specialty areas) have 15 alternate completion questions available for each exam, which can be substituted for the last 15 questions of the exam. These alternate questions concentrate on word elements and abbreviations.

The instructor may choose to use the exams exactly as provided in the instructor's manual, or may prefer to select questions from several exams, combining them into an entirely new exam that would fit the sample course syllabus format. Answers for all chapter exams are included at the end of the *Instructor's Manual.*

Exams can also be used as questions for the *Medical Terminology Challenge* game that is suggested in the section on classroom activities.

SAMPLE COURSE SYLLABUS

A sample course syllabus has been provided. This syllabus allows for teaching this textbook over the course of two semesters.

COURSE SYLLABUS
FIRST SEMESTER
(Two-semester Sequence)

Days	Topic	Chapter	# Contact Hours
1	Review of Course Syllabus and Class Requirements. Review of Text Format and How to Use the Text.		1
2-3	Word Building Rules	1	2
4-6	Prefixes	2	3
7-9	Suffixes	3	3
10	**EXAM I: Chapters 1-3**		1
11-13	Whole Body Terms	4	3
14-18	Integumentary System	5	5
19	**EXAM II: Chapters 4-5**		1
20-23	Skeletal System	6	4
24-27	Muscles and Joints	7	4
28	**EXAM III: Chapters 6-7**		1
29-33	Nervous System	8	5
34-38	Blood and Lymphatic System	9	5
39	**EXAM IV: Chapters 8-9**		1
40-43	Cardiovascular System	10	4
44-47	Respiratory System	11	4
48	**EXAM V: Chapters 10-11**		

COURSE SYLLABUS
SECOND SEMESTER
(Two-semester Sequence)

Days	Topic	Chapter	# Contact Hours
1	Review of Course Syllabus and Class Requirements. Review of Word Building Rules		1
2-5	Digestive System	12	4
6-9	Endocrine System	13	4
10	**EXAM I: Chapters 12-13**		1
11-14	Special Senses	14	4
15-17	Urinary System	15	3
18	**EXAM II: Chapters 14-15**		1
19-21	Male Reproductive System	16	3
22-25	Female Reproductive System	17	4
26	**EXAM III: Chapters 16-17**		1
27-30	Obstetrics	18	4
31-33	Child Health	19	3
34	**EXAM IV: Chapters 18-19**		1
35-37	Radiology and Diagnostic Imaging	20	3
38-40	Oncology	21	3
41	**EXAM V: Chapters 20-21**		1
42-44	Pharmacology	22	3
45-47	Mental Health	23	3
48	**EXAM VI: Chapters 22-23**		

SUGGESTED CLASSROOM ACTIVITIES

The classroom activites listed in this section can be applied to any of the chapter topics within the text. The instructor may select the ones that best fit the time frame for the particular subject.

1. **LIBRARY TOUR**
   Each student enrolled in a medical terminology course should possess a knowledge of available library resources. A good way to begin a course is with a tour of the campus library, familiarizing the students with the location of medical textbooks, magazines, reference books, use of the Internet to research materials, audiovisual materials available, and the procedures necessary for securing information. This could be scheduled for the first or second day of class.

2. **DICTIONARY REVIEW**
   A general review of the proper way to use the medical dictionary is a good way to begin the course. Students should be guided through pronouncing sounds appropriately. For example, the "ph" sound, which sounds like an "f"; the "ch" sound, which sounds like a "k"; the hard "g" and the soft "g" sounds; the hard "c" and the soft "c" sounds, etc. The instructor could pronounce the sounds aloud for the students and have them repeat them aloud as a group.

   Throughout the textbook, there are various chapter exercises that encourage students to use their medical dictionary. These could be selected ahead of time and assigned to ensure the use of the medical dictionary.

3. **NEWSPAPER/MAGAZINE/INTERNET ARTICLES**
   When studying the various body systems, extra credit can be given to students who bring in newspaper, magazine, or internet articles that relate to the particular system being studied. This is a good way to keep the class informed of some of the most up-to-date medical information in the news.

   The instructor might prefer to assign topics for the student to research on any one of the pathological conditions being studied in the assigned chapter and write a one-page report for extra credit.

4. **PATHOPHYSIOLOGY SHEETS**
   If this course is the only exposure to pathology/symptomatology that the students will receive, the instructor might consider having the students complete "Pathophysiology Sheets" for each unit. Specific topics can be assigned, or the student could pick the particular pathological condition of choice, complete additional reading on the topic, and write a one-page report on the topic using the format included. You may wish to copy the *Pathophysiology Sheet Template* form on page ix for students to use.

5. **CREATE A STORY**
   If time permits the use of alternate learning methods, a fun—and challenging—way to reinforce the meaning of medical words and the word elements is to have the students create a story using the words and word elements from an assigned chapter. The story must have continuity, must have a title, must use as many words and word elements as possible, and must be appropriate for reading aloud. A prize could be given for the student(s) using the most medical words and word elements from the chapter. If preferred, the instructor can supply a list for use by the students, to provide a little more structure to the project.

   The medical words and word elements are to be substituted for words in the story, followed by a blank space. As the student reads the story to the class, the class members will fill in the blanks with the appropriate definitions, completing the meaning in the story. For example,

   "Pierre was a glyc/o ______________ little old man. He
   (sweet)
   suffered from cryptorchidism ______________________________."
   (undescended testicles)

   The instructor can provide the students with the *Create a Story* sample on page xi of this manual to use as a guide when creating their stories. If time permits, the instructor can collect the stories in advance, transfer them to a transparency sheet, and project them onto a screen for viewing by the entire class. This is a good way to promote class participation—and its fun!

Pathophysiology Sheet

STUDENT'S NAME: ______________________________ COURSE: ______________

DATE: ____ CHAPTER: _____________

TOPIC: ____

Description of Condition:

Characteristics of the Condition:

Treatments:

Source:

Create-A-Story
(Based on Chapter 10: Cardiovascular System)

The Story of Elmo Strange

Elmo Strange was a ather/o ______________________ little old man who owned a sock factory. He lived end/o ______________________ the small town of Yorkshire. The only problem that Elmo had was that he had an megal/o ______________________ opinion of himself.

Elmo's employees felt that he had a cold cardi/o ______________________ when it came to paying them or giving raises. He expected his employees to keep an accurate gram ______________________ of every sock made or discarded. Elmo refused to raise salaries of his employees, which were already low. When he said "NO," he expected not a ech/o ______________________ to be uttered by anyone! It was enough to cause the employees to have spasms of the arteri/o ______________________ . After all, it took a lot of my/o ______________________ to run the machines that knitted the socks. The working hours were so long that the employees complained of fatigue ______________________ and edema ______________________ of the feet from standing on the cement floor so long.

One day during an electr/o ______________________ storm, Elmo's sock factory caught on fire! Elmo experienced nausea ______________________ , anxiety ______________________ , and palpitations ______________________ when he thought he might lose everything! Thanks to the quick action of his employees the fire was quickly extinguished. They saved the sock factory!

Elmo's pallor ______________________ disappeared. He was so happy to have his factory saved. He was so pleased with his employees that he gave everyone a very big raise! The employees were thrilled! They then realized that Elmo Strange had a "cardi/o" ______________________ after all!

Answers to Create-A-Story
(Based on Chapter 10: Cardiovascular System)

ather/o	fatty
end/o	within
megal/o	enlarged
gram	record
ech/o	sound
arteri/o	arteries
my/o	muscle
fatigue	a feeling of weakness
edema	swelling
electr/o	electrical
nausea	an uncomfortable feeling that the contents of the stomach will be returned through the mouth
anxiety	an uneasy, nervous feeling
palpitations	unusually rapid, strong beating of the heart
pallor	paleness of the skin
cardi/o	heart

6. **VOCABULARY DRILLS**

Vocabulary drills are a great way to reinforce the spelling of medical terms. If the audiotapes that accompany this textbook are available, the student can complete this assignment outside of class or as part of a class project. The tape should be played and the student could be instructed to key in the words on a computer as they are pronounced. If a computer is not available, the student can write the words as they are pronounced on the tape. If students are unsure about the spelling of the word, they can refer to a medical dictionary for necessary corrections. The goal for the student is to complete the list, check it by the dictionary for accurate spelling, and submit a correctly spelled list to the instructor. This could count for bonus points.

Students should be encouraged to rewrite any misspelled words a minimum of 3 times, to reinforce the accurate spelling of the word. This may seem a little elementary, but it works.

7. **MEDICAL TERMINOLOGY "CHALLENGE"**

If computers are available for classroom use and *Delmar's Medical Terminology Challenge* game is installed on the computers, the instructor can divide the class into teams for an assigned period of time (15 minutes or so) and allow the teams to play "Medical Terminology Challenge" on the computer. You can order *Delmar's Medical Terminology Challenge* by calling 1-800-347-7707. The ISBN order number is 0-8273-6675-2. At the end of the assigned time period, the team with the highest score wins a prize. Halloween is a good time to play this game, with the winning team earning a bag of Halloween candy as a prize. A consolation prize of a piece of gum or candy can be given to all participants.

If computers are not accessible to the class, a "Medical Terminology Challenge Board" can be drawn and made into a transparency using the guide on page xii. This can then be used by projecting the format onto a screen in the class, with the instructor calling the words/definitions for the challenge. When the category is used, the instructor can cover the space on the transparency. A sample Medical Terminology Challenge board format is provided. The instructor can use the chapter exam questions, included in this manual, for game questions when playing *Medical Terminology Challenge.*

Medical Terminology Challenge

Word Elements	Abbreviations	Conditions	Treatments	Definitions
$100	$100	$100	$100	$100
$200	$200	$200	$200	$200
$300	$300	$300	$300	$300
$400	$400	$400	$400	$400
$500	$500	$500	$500	$500

8. **WORD ELEMENT REVIEW SHEETS**
The word element review sheets can be used for independent study or as "warm-ups" before beginnning a class. Samples are included in each chapter of this manual.

9. **THREE STRIKES, YOU'RE OUT!**
This game is played using words from the chapter being studied at the time. The instructor should make a master list of words to be used in the game. You may wish to select words from the written and Audio Review list at the end of the textbook chapters.

Divide the class into teams, with 4-5 members per team, depending on the class size. Designate a score keeper for each team. The object of this game is to earn the highest number of points within the designated time period.

Items needed for the game will include a watch with a second hand for timing, a box or a bag, large enough to mix the game cards well, and a package of blank 3" x 5" index cards for writing the letters for the game. The instructor will make 7 cards with one letter on each card as illustrated below.

Card # 1: VOWEL
Card # 2: VOWEL
Card # 3: "X"
Card # 4: "X"
Card # 5: "X"
Card # 6: CONSONANT
Card # 7: CONSONANT

The instructor should draw the appropriate number of spaces on the board to match the number of letters in the word; place all 7 cards in the box and mix them well.

One representative from a team will play at a time. The representing team member will draw a card. If the card has "Consonant", the team member can guess a consonant. If the consonant guessed appears in the word, the instructor will write the consonant in the appropriate place(s). If the card has "Vowel", the team member can guess a vowel. If the vowel guessed appears in the word, the instructor will write the vowel in the appropriate place(s). ***NOTE:*** *The team member, only, can guess the consonants and/or vowels, but the team as a whole can guess the word.*

After a consonant or a vowel is placed in the appropriate space, the team has 30 seconds to confer and guess the word, if they think they know it. If a guess is not made, another card is drawn. Play continues until the team either correctly guesses the word, which awards the team 20 points; the team incorrectly guesses the word and the turn is over; or the team member draws 3 strikes and the play is over.

The representing team member can earn 5 bonus points for the team if he/she correctly defines the word on the board.

Each time a new team member takes a turn, the instructor places the appropriate number of spaces on the board for the new word, mixes the cards again, and play continues. At the end of the designated time period, the points are tallied and the winning team is determined.

10. **FLASH CARDS**
Flash cards can be used to review the various word elements in the chapters. It is suggested that the students make their own flash cards on index cards. The student can use codes in the upper right corner of each card to identify the word element. Place the word element on one side of the card and the definition on the other side of the card. Two sample cards (front and back) are illustrated below.

CF	CF
rhin/o	**nose**
Card Front	Card Back
S	S
-itis	**inflammation**
Card Front	Card Back

The codes for the upper right corner of each card front and back should be as follows: **P** = prefix, **S** = suffix, **CF** = combining form.

After making the flash cards, the student should review them two ways: from the word element to the definition, and from the definition to the word element.

a. The student should stack the cards with the word elements "face up," define the word element and turn the card over to check for accuracy.
b. If the student's answer is correct, place the card in a discard stack.
c. If the student's answer is incorrect, place the card at the bottom of the stack of cards to review again.
d. The student should make a list of any word elements missed and should write each element, along with its definition, a minimum of 3 times to reinforce the meaning and the word element.
e. Students should review the stack of cards until they can complete the entire set without error.
f. Upon completing the review of the word element side, turn the stack of cards over with the definitions "face up." The student should identify the word element based upon the definition and turn the card over to check for accuracy.
g. Repeat steps b through e.
h. Once students have mastered the word elements, flash cards can be used with the complete word on one side and the definition on the other side. With this method, two students can work together. One student will quiz the other by flashing the "definition" and having the other student identify the word that appears on the back of the card. If the answer is correct, the student can ask his or her partner the following about the word:
    - Spell the word.
    - Use the word in a sentence.
i. If the student cannot spell the word correctly, he/she should write the word a minimum of 3 times to reinforce the correct spelling.

TRANSCRIPTION WORD LIST EXERCISES

At the end of each chapter is an audiocassette review list. These words can be used as transcription review exercises to strengthen the student's listening, keying, proofing, and spelling skills. This can be accomplished in one of the following ways:

- The instructor may prefer to call the words aloud, from the lists, for students to key in on the computer as they hear them.
- Students can listen to the words on the *Comprehensive Medical Teminology* audiocassettes, if available, and can transcribe the assigned number of words (i.e., the first 25 words) for a quiz grade or extra credit.
- Students without the *Comprehensive Medical Terminology* audiocassettes can record the assigned words on their own tape recorders at home and play them back later for transcribing.

CROSSOVER GUIDE

TOPICS / SYSTEMS	DELMAR Davis-Jones	SAUNDERS Chabner 5th edition	F.A. DAVIS Gylys/Wedding 3rd edition
Word Building Rules	Ch. 1	Ch. 1	Ch. 1
Prefixes	Ch. 2	Ch. 4	Ch. 4
Suffixes	Ch. 3	Ch. 3	Ch. 2 & 3
Whole Body Terms	Ch. 4	Ch. 2	Ch. 5
Integumentary	Ch. 5	Ch. 16	Ch. 6
Skeletal	Ch. 6	Ch.15	Ch. 11
Muscles and Joints	Ch. 7	Ch. 15	Ch. 11
Nervous	Ch. 8	Ch. 10	Ch. 15
Blood and Lymphatic	Ch. 9	Ch.13 & 14	Ch. 10
Cardiovascular	Ch. 10	Ch. 11	Ch. 9
Respiratory	Ch. 11	Ch. 12	Ch. 8
Digestive	Ch. 12	Ch. 5	Ch. 7
Endocrine	Ch. 13	Ch. 18	Ch. 14
Special Senses (Eye and Ear)	Ch. 14	Ch. 17	Ch. 16
Urinary	Ch. 15	Ch. 7	Ch. 12
Male Reproductive	Ch. 16	Ch. 9	Ch. 12
Female Reproductive	Ch. 17	Ch. 8	Ch. 12
Obstetrics	Ch. 18	------	Ch. 13
Child Health	Ch. 19	------	------
Radiology/Diagnostic Imaging	Ch. 20	Ch. 20	------
Oncology	Ch. 21	Ch. 19	Ch. 16
Pharmacology	Ch. 22	Ch. 21	------
Mental Health	Ch. 23	Ch. 22	------

SUPPLEMENTARY MATERIALS

Practice CD-ROM

Free student practice software is packaged with each textbook. The software is designed to offer the students additional practice with terminology by providing: diagram exercises; review exercises in choice of completion, matching, multiple choice, true and false questions; as well as several games and practice tests. Students can track their progress through the chapters. Additional software documentation is included on pages 209–216 of this manual as well as in the *How to Use the Practice CD-ROM* section on pages xx–xxi of the textbook.

Audiotapes

(Available in text/tape value package ISBN 0-7668-9494-1 or with duplication rights ISBN 0-7668-0496-8)

Two 90-minute audiotapes accompany this text and have been developed to allow students to listen to each term and repeat it aloud for pronunciation practice. Students may also use the tapes to listen to the terms while they follow along with the *Written and Audio Terminology Review* section of body system and specialty chapters.

Computerized Test Bank

(ISBN 0-7668-0497-6)

The computerized test bank includes over 1000 questions with answers and is available in Windows format (3.5" disk) to easily create a variety of testing materials with your personal computer. You can even add your own questions to the test bank.

Delmar's Medical Terminology Image Library

(ISBN 0-7668-0492-5)

This CD-ROM includes over 600 graphic files that can be incorporated into a PowerPoint, Microsoft® Word, or WordPerfect® presentation, used directly off the CD-ROM in a classroom presentation, or used to make color transparencies. The Image Library is organized around body systems and medical specialties. The library will include various anatomy, physiology, and pathology graphics of different complexity. Instructors can search and select the graphics that best apply to their teaching situation. This is an ideal resource to enhance your teaching presentation of medical terminology or anatomy and physiology.

Delmar's Audiotape Set for Medical Terminology

(ISBN 0-7668-0491-7 duplication rights included)

These eight, 90-minute audiotapes include the pronunciation of the term, definition of the word parts and term, and examples of terms used in context. The audiotapes are organized by body system for ease of use. The audiotapes include common pronunciation variations for terms (where applicable) to alert the student to differences. An On-line Companion will be available to produce a hard copy of the taped content for students to follow along.

SUGGESTED SOFTWARE PRODUCTS

Delmar's Medical Terminology Challenge Software, 1996, by John Pucillo, Delmar Publishers, Albany, New York

A fun, interactive way to assess and reinforce understanding of word-building principles, common word elements, and body system terminology. Very affordable!

Flash! Medical Terminology Flashcard Software, 1996, Delmar Publishers, Albany, New York

This 500 flashcard-type question and answer program is designed to help users learn and retain medical terms, word combinations, and medications quickly and easily, with or without a timer.

Medical Terminology CD-ROM: A Visual Guide, 1997, Delmar Publishers, Albany, New York

This interactive CD-ROM program presents terminology in modules that include screens on origins, anatomy, word building, context, procedures, technology, health care issues and more. The CD-ROM provides the users with basic knowledge of medical terminology, categorized by body system and can be used with any text or independently. Both Institutional and Individual Versions are available.

COMING... JANUARY 1999!

Delmar's Medical Terminology CD-ROM (ISBN 0-7668-0979-X)

New CD-ROM developed around medical terms and organized around word-building, body systems, and specialties sections. This highly interactive CD includes videos of actual procedures (no talking heads) and 50 animations of dynamic processes. Interactive activities in a fun format are included as well as assessment tests for each section.

CHAPTER REVIEW SHEETS

The review sheets are grouped together in this section in chapter order. There are no review sheets for Chapter 1 since it concentrates on word building rules. The instructor will note, however, that Chapter 1 is referred to many times throughout the text when emphasis is placed on word building rules. The learner will be reminded often to refer to the chapter on word building rules.

The remaining chapters of the text each have review sheets available that can be used as classroom drills or as assigned work outside of class. Each chapter has one or more review sheets that challenge the learner's thought processes to move from the word element to the definition, and one or more review sheets that challenge the learner's thought processes to move from the definition to the word element.

The review sheets can also be used to drill the learners in the correct pronunciation of the words. The instructor should pronounce the word elements first and the learners should respond with the same pronunciation (as a group).

CHAPTER 2: PREFIXES
CHAPTER REVIEW SHEET 1

INSTRUCTIONS: Write the meaning of each word element in the space provided. Check your answers by referring to the word element review within the chapter.

WORD ELEMENT TO DEFINITION

WORD ELEMENT	DEFINITION
1. a-	
2. ab-	
3. ad-	
4. alb-	
5. ambi-	
6. an-	
7. ante-	
8. anti-	
9. auto-	
10. bi-	
11. bio-	
12. brady-	
13. circum-	
14. con-	
15. contra-	
16. de-	
17. dis-	
18. dys-	
19. ecto-	
20. endo-	

Number Correct_____X 05 Points Per Correct Answer: Your Score_____%

CHAPTER 2: PREFIXES
CHAPTER REVIEW SHEET 2

INSTRUCTIONS: Write the appropriate word element for each definition given. Place your answer in the space provided. Check your answers by referring to the word element review within the chapter.

DEFINITION TO WORD ELEMENT

DEFINITION	WORD ELEMENT
1. without, away from	
2. from, away from	
3. toward, increase	
4. white	
5. both, both sides	
6. without, not (different word from #1)	
7. before, in front	
8. against	
9. self	
10. two, double	
11. life	
12. slow	
13. around	
14. together, with	
15. against (different word from #8)	
16. down, from	
17. free of, to undo	
18. bad, difficult	
19. outside	
20. within	

Number Correct_____X 05 Points Per Correct Answer: Your Score_____%

CHAPTER 2: PREFIXES
CHAPTER REVIEW SHEET 3

INSTRUCTIONS: Write the meaning of each word element in the space provided. Check your answers by referring to the word element review within the chapter.

WORD ELEMENT TO DEFINITION

WORD ELEMENT	DEFINITION
1. epi-	
2. eu-	
3. ex-	
4. extra-	
5. hemi-	
6. homeo-	
7. homo-	
8. hydro-	
9. hyper-	
10. hypo-	
11. idio-	
12. in-	
13. infra-	
14. inter-	
15. intra-	
16. juxta-	
17. meta-	
18. milli-	
19. mono-	
20. multi-	

Number Correct_____X 05 Points Per Correct Answer: Your Score_____%

CHAPTER 2: PREFIXES
CHAPTER REVIEW SHEET 4

INSTRUCTIONS: Write the appropriate word element for each definition given. Place your answer in the space provided. Check your answers by referring to the word element review within the chapter.

DEFINITION TO WORD ELEMENT

DEFINITION	WORD ELEMENT
1. upon, over	
2. good, normal	
3. out, away from	
4. outside of, beyond	
5. half	
6. likeness, same	
7. same (different word from #6)	
8. water	
9. excessive	
10. less than, under	
11. individual	
12. in, within, not	
13. beneath, under	
14. between	
15. within	
16. near, beside	
17. change, after	
18. one-thousandth	
19. one, single	
20. many	

Number Correct_____X 05 Points Per Correct Answer: Your Score_____%

CHAPTER 2: PREFIXES
CHAPTER REVIEW SHEET 5

INSTRUCTIONS: Write the meaning of each word element in the space provided. Check your answers by referring to the word element review within the chapter.

WORD ELEMENT TO DEFINITION

WORD ELEMENT	DEFINITION
1. non-	
2. pan-	
3. para-	
4. per-	
5. peri-	
6. poly-	
7. post-	
8. pre-	
9. primi-	
10. pseudo-	
11. retro-	
12. semi-	
13. sub-	
14. supra-	
15. sym-	
16. tachy-	
17. trans-	
18. tri-	
19. uni-	
20. xero-	

Number Correct_____X 05 Points Per Correct Answer: Your Score_____%

CHAPTER 2: PREFIXES
CHAPTER REVIEW SHEET 6

INSTRUCTIONS: Write the appropriate word element for each definition given. Place your answer in the space provided. Check your answers by referring to the word element review within the chapter.

DEFINITION TO WORD ELEMENT

DEFINITION	WORD ELEMENT
1. not	
2. all	
3. near, beside	
4. through	
5. around	
6. many, much	
7. after, behind	
8. before, in front	
9. first	
10. false	
11. backward, behind	
12. half	
13. under, below	
14. above, over	
15. joined, together	
16. rapid	
17. across, through	
18. three	
19. one	
20. dry	

Number Correct_____X 05 Points Per Correct Answer: Your Score_____%

CHAPTER 3: SUFFIXES
CHAPTER REVIEW SHEET 1

INSTRUCTIONS: Write the meaning of each word element in the space provided. Check your answers by referring to the word element review within the chapter.

WORD ELEMENT TO DEFINITION

WORD ELEMENT	DEFINITION
1. -ac, -al	
2. -ad	
3. -algesia	
4. -algia	
5. -ate	
6. -blast	
7. -cele	
8. -centesis	
9. -cide	
10. -clasis	
11. -cyte	
12. -dynia	
13. -e, -a	
14. -ectasia	
15. -ectomy	
16. -emia	
17. -er	
18. -esis	
19. -genesis	
20. -gram	

Number Correct_____X 05 Points Per Correct Answer: Your Score_____%

CHAPTER 3: SUFFIXES
CHAPTER REVIEW SHEET 2

INSTRUCTIONS: Write the appropriate word element for each definition given. Place your answer in the space provided. Check your answers by referring to the word element review within the chapter.

DEFINITION TO WORD ELEMENT

DEFINITION	WORD ELEMENT
1. pertaining to	
2. toward	
3. sensitivity to pain	
4. pain	
5. something that	
6. immature, embryonic	
7. herniation	
8. surgical puncture	
9. to kill	
10. crushing or breaking up	
11. cell	
12. pain (other than #4)	
13. noun ending	
14. stretching, dilatation	
15. surgical removal	
16. blood condition	
17. one who	
18. condition of	
19. generating, formation	
20. record or picture	

Number Correct_____X 05 Points Per Correct Answer: Your Score_____%

CHAPTER 3: SUFFIXES
CHAPTER REVIEW SHEET 3

INSTRUCTIONS: Write the meaning of each word element in the space provided. Check your answers by referring to the word element review within the chapter.

WORD ELEMENT TO DEFINITION

WORD ELEMENT	DEFINITION
1. -graph	
2. -graphy	
3. -ia	
4. -ion	
5. -ist	
6. -itis	
7. -lepsy	
8. -lith	
9. -logy	
10. -logist	
11. -lysis	
12. -mania	
13. -megaly	
14. -meter	
15. -metry	
16. -oid	
17. -ole	
18. -oma	
19. -opia	
20. -osis	

Number Correct_____X 05 Points Per Correct Answer: Your Score_____%

CHAPTER 3: SUFFIXES
CHAPTER REVIEW SHEET 4

INSTRUCTIONS: Write the appropriate word element for each definition given. Place your answer in the space provided. Check your answers by referring to the word element review within the chapter.

DEFINITION TO WORD ELEMENT

DEFINITION	WORD ELEMENT
1. instrument used to record	
2. process of recording	
3. condition	
4. action	
5. one who (a specialist in a field of study)	
6. inflammation	
7. seizure	
8. stone	
9. the study of	
10. one who specializes in the study of	
11. destruction	
12. madness	
13. enlargement	
14. an instrument used to measure	
15. the process of measuring	
16. resembling	
17. small or little	
18. tumor	
19. visual condition	
20. condition (other than #3)	

Number Correct_____X 05 Points Per Correct Answer: Your Score_____%

CHAPTER 3: SUFFIXES
CHAPTER REVIEW SHEET 5

INSTRUCTIONS: Write the meaning of each word element in the space provided. Check your answers by referring to the word element review within the chapter.

WORD ELEMENT TO DEFINITION

WORD ELEMENT	DEFINITION
1. -pathy	
2. -penia	
3. -pexy	
4. -philia	
5. -phobia	
6. -plasty	
7. -plegia	
8. -pnea	
9. -ptosis	
10. -rrhagia	
11. -rrhaphy	
12. -rrhea	
13. -rrhexis	
14. -scope	
15. -stomy	
16. -tomy	
17. -tripsy	
18. -uria	
19. -stasis	
20. -scopy	

Number Correct_____X 05 Points Per Correct Answer: Your Score_____%

CHAPTER 3: SUFFIXES
CHAPTER REVIEW SHEET 6

INSTRUCTIONS: Write the appropriate word element for each definition given. Place your answer in the space provided. Check your answers by referring to the word element review within the chapter.

DEFINITION TO WORD ELEMENT

DEFINITION	WORD ELEMENT
1. disease	
2. decrease in, deficiency	
3. surgical fixation	
4. attracted to	
5. abnormal fear	
6. surgical repair	
7. paralysis, stroke	
8. breathing	
9. drooping, prolapse	
10. excessive flow, bursting forth	
11. suturing	
12. drainage, flow	
13. rupture	
14. instrument used to view	
15. creation of a new opening	
16. incision into	
17. crushing	
18. a characteristic of urine	
19. stopping or controlling	
20. the process of viewing with an instrument	

Number Correct_____ X 05 Points Per Correct Answer: Your Score_____%

CHAPTER 4: WHOLE BODY TERMS
CHAPTER REVIEW SHEET 1

INSTRUCTIONS: Write the meaning of each word element in the space provided. Check your answers by referring to the word element review within the chapter.

WORD ELEMENT TO DEFINITION

WORD ELEMENT	DEFINITION
1. abdomin/o	
2. anter/o	
3. cervic/o	
4. coccyg/o	
5. crani/o	
6. cyt/o	
7. dors/o	
8. umbilic/o	
9. thorac/o	
10. hist/o	
11. ili/o	
12. inguin/o	
13. sacr/o	
14. later/o	
15. medi/o	
16. nucle/o	
17. pelv/i	
18. proxim/o	
19. ventr/o	
20. viscer/o	

Number Correct_____X 05 Points Per Correct Answer: Your Score_____%

CHAPTER 4: WHOLE BODY TERMS
CHAPTER REVIEW SHEET 2

INSTRUCTIONS: Write the appropriate word element for each definition given. Place your answer in the space provided. Check your answers by referring to the word element review within the chapter.

DEFINITION TO WORD ELEMENT

DEFINITION	WORD ELEMENT
1. abdomen	
2. front	
3. neck	
4. coccyx	
5. skull, cranium	
6. cell	
7. back	
8. navel	
9. chest	
10. tissue	
11. ilium	
12. groin	
13. sacrum	
14. side	
15. middle	
16. nucleus	
17. pelvis	
18. near	
19. belly, front side	
20. internal organs	

Number Correct_____X 05 Points Per Correct Answer: Your Score_____%

CHAPTER 5: INTEGUMENTARY SYSTEM
CHAPTER REVIEW SHEET 1

INSTRUCTIONS: Write the meaning of each word element in the space provided. Check your answers by referring to the word element review within the chapter.

WORD ELEMENT TO DEFINITION

WORD ELEMENT	DEFINITION
1. adip/o	
2. cutane/o	
3. derm/o	
4. dermat/o	
5. hidr/o	
6. kerat/o	
7. lip/o	
8. erythr/o	
9. leuk/o	
10. melan/o	
11. xanth/o	
12. myc/o	
13. onych/o	
14. pil/o	
15. scler/o	
16. squam/o	
17. trich/o	
18. xer/o	
19. ichthy/o	
20. cauter/o	

Number Correct_____X 05 Points Per Correct Answer: Your Score_____%

CHAPTER 5: INTEGUMENTARY SYSTEM
CHAPTER REVIEW SHEET 2

INSTRUCTIONS: Write the appropriate word element for each definition given. Place your answer in the space provided. Check your answers by referring to the word element review within the chapter.

DEFINITION TO WORD ELEMENT

DEFINITION	WORD ELEMENT
1. pertaining to fat	
2. skin	
3. skin (other than #2)	
4. skin (other than #3)	
5. sweat	
6. horny	
7. fat	
8. red	
9. white	
10. black	
11. yellow	
12. fungus	
13. nails	
14. hair	
15. hard	
16. scales	
17. hair (other than #14)	
18. dryness	
19. fish	
20. burn	

Number Correct_____X 05 Points Per Correct Answer: Your Score_____%

CHAPTER 6: SKELETAL SYSTEM
CHAPTER REVIEW SHEET 1

INSTRUCTIONS: Write the meaning of each word element in the space provided. Check your answers by referring to the word element review within the chapter.

WORD ELEMENT TO DEFINITION

WORD ELEMENT	DEFINITION
1. acetabul/o	
2. blast/o	
3. calc/i	
4. calcane/o	
5. carp/o	
6. -clast	
7. clavicul/o	
8. coccyg/o	
9. cost/o	
10. crani/o	
11. femor/o	
12. fibul/o	
13. gen/o	
14. humer/o	
15. ili/o	
16. ischi/o	
17. kyph/o	
18. lamin/o	
19. lumb/o	
20. -malacia	

Number Correct_____X 05 Points Per Correct Answer: Your Score_____%

CHAPTER 6: SKELETAL SYSTEM
CHAPTER REVIEW SHEET 2

INSTRUCTIONS: Write the appropriate word element for each definition given. Place your answer in the space provided. Check your answers by referring to the word element review within the chapter.

DEFINITION TO WORD ELEMENT

DEFINITION	WORD ELEMENT
1. acetabulum	
2. embryonic	
3. calcium	
4. heel bone	
5. wrist	
6. to break (suffix)	
7. collar bone	
8. coccyx	
9. ribs	
10. skull	
11. femur	
12. fibula	
13. produce	
14. humerus	
15. ilium	
16. ischium	
17. humpback	
18. lamina	
19. lower back	
20. softening (suffix)	

Number Correct_____X 05 Points Per Correct Answer: Your Score_____%

CHAPTER 6: SKELETAL SYSTEM
CHAPTER REVIEW SHEET 3

INSTRUCTIONS: Write the meaning of each word element in the space provided. Check your answers by referring to the word element review within the chapter.

WORD ELEMENT TO DEFINITION

WORD ELEMENT	DEFINITION
1. mastoid/o	
2. maxill/o	
3. metacarp/o	
4. metatars/o	
5. myel/o	
6. olecran/o	
7. orth/o	
8. oste/o	
9. patell/o	
10. pelv/i	
11. phalang/o	
12. -physis	
13. -porosis	
14. pub/o	
15. rach/i	
16. scoli/o	
17. spondyl/o	
18. radi/o	
19. scapul/o	
20. tars/o	

Number Correct_____X 05 Points Per Correct Answer: Your Score_____%

CHAPTER 6: SKELETAL SYSTEM
CHAPTER REVIEW SHEET 4

INSTRUCTIONS: Write the appropriate word element for each definition given. Place your answer in the space provided. Check your answers by referring to the word element review within the chapter.

DEFINITION TO WORD ELEMENT

DEFINITION	WORD ELEMENT
1. mastoid process	
2. upper jaw	
3. hand bones	
4. foot bones	
5. bone marrow	
6. elbow	
7. straight	
8. bone	
9. kneecap	
10. pelvis	
11. fingers, toes	
12. growth, growing (suffix)	
13. passage or pore (suffix)	
14. pubis	
15. spinal column	
16. crooked, bent	
17. vertebrae	
18. radius	
19. shoulder blade	
20. ankle bones	

Number Correct_____X 05 Points Per Correct Answer Your Score_____%

CHAPTER 7: MUSCLES AND JOINTS
CHAPTER REVIEW SHEET 1

INSTRUCTIONS: Write the meaning of each word element in the space provided. Check your answers by referring to the word element review within the chapter.

WORD ELEMENT TO DEFINITION

WORD ELEMENT	DEFINITION
1. bucc/o	
2. fasci/o	
3. fibr/o	
4. leiomy/o	
5. my/o	
6. pector/o, thorac/o	
7. rhabdomy/o	
8. tri-	
9. troph/o	
10. ankyl/o	
11. arthr/o	
12. articul/o	
13. burs/o	
14. ligament/o	
15. oste/o	
16. ten/o	
17. tendin/o	
18. tend/o	
19. electr/o	
20. dors/o	

Number Correct_____X 05 Points Per Correct Answer: Your Score_____%

CHAPTER 7: MUSCLES AND JOINTS
CHAPTER REVIEW SHEET 2

INSTRUCTIONS: Write the appropriate word element for each definition given. Place your answer in the space provided. Check your answers by referring to the word element review within the chapter.

DEFINITION TO WORD ELEMENT

DEFINITION	WORD ELEMENT
1. cheek	
2. band of fibrous tissue	
3. fiber	
4. smooth muscle	
5. muscle	
6. pertaining to the chest	
7. striated muscle	
8. three (prefix)	
9. development	
10. stiff	
11. joint	
12. joint (other than #11)	
13. bursa	
14. ligament	
15. bone	
16. tendon	
17. tendon (other than #16)	
18. tendon (other than #17)	
19. electricity	
20. back	

Number Correct_____X 05 Points Per Correct Answer: Your Score_____%

CHAPTER 8: NERVOUS SYSTEM CHAPTER REVIEW SHEET 1

INSTRUCTIONS: Write the meaning of each word element in the space provided. Check your answers by referring to the word element review within the chapter.

WORD ELEMENT TO DEFINITION

WORD ELEMENT	DEFINITION
1. cerebell/o	
2. cerebr/o	
3. encephal/o	
4. esthesi/o, -esthesia	
5. gli/o	
6. kinesi/o, -kinesia	
7. myel/o	
8. narc/o	
9. neur/o	
10. ton/o	
11. ventricul/o	
12. -sthenia	
13. thec/o	
14. -phasia	
15. -lexia	
16. -lepsy	
17. mening/o	
18. narc/o	
19. alges/o, -algesia	
20. -algia	

Number Correct_____X 05 Points Per Correct Answer: Your Score_____%

CHAPTER 8: NERVOUS SYSTEM
CHAPTER REVIEW SHEET 2

INSTRUCTIONS: Write the appropriate word element for each definition given. Place your answer in the space provided. Check your answers by referring to the word element review within the chapter.

DEFINITION TO WORD ELEMENT

DEFINITION	WORD ELEMENT
1. cerebellum	
2. cerebrum	
3. brain	
4. sensation or feeling	
5. pertaining to neuroglia cells	
6. movement	
7. spinal cord or bone marrow	
8. sleep	
9. nerve	
10. tension	
11. ventricle	
12. strength (suffix)	
13. sheath	
14. speech (suffix)	
15. reading (suffix)	
16. seizure (suffix)	
17. meninges	
18. sleep	
19. sensitivity to pain	
20. pain (suffix)	

Number Correct_____X 05 Points Per Correct Answer: Your Score_____%

CHAPTER 9: BLOOD & LYMPHATIC SYSTEM
CHAPTER REVIEW SHEET 1

INSTRUCTIONS: Write the meaning of each word element in the space provided. Check your answers by referring to the word element review within the chapter.

WORD ELEMENT TO DEFINITION

WORD ELEMENT	DEFINITION
1. agglutin/o	
2. anis/o	
3. bas/o	
4. blast/o, -blast	
5. chrom/o	
6. coagul/o	
7. cyt/o	
8. -emia	
9. eosin/o	
10. erythr/o	
11. -globin	
12. hem/o, hemat/o	
13. hem/o, hemat/o	
14. kary/o	
15. morph/o	
16. phag/o, -phage	
17. poikil/o	
18. sider/o	
19. spher/o	
20. thromb/o	

Number Correct_____X 05 Points Per Correct Answer: Your Score_____%

CHAPTER 9: BLOOD & LYMPHATIC SYSTEM
CHAPTER REVIEW SHEET 2

INSTRUCTIONS: Write the appropriate word element for each definition given. Place your answer in the space provided. Check your answers by referring to the word element review within the chapter.

DEFINITION TO WORD ELEMENT

DEFINITION	WORD ELEMENT
1. to clump	
2. unequal	
3. base	
4. embryonic state of development	
5. color	
6. clotting	
7. cell	
8. blood condition (suffix)	
9. red, rosy	
10. red	
11. containing protein (suffix)	
12. blood	
13. blood (other than #12)	
14. nucleus	
15. form, shape	
16. to eat	
17. varied, irregular	
18. iron	
19. round; sphere	
20. clot	

Number Correct_____X 05 Points Per Correct Answer: Your Score_____%

CHAPTER 10: CARDIOVASCULAR SYSTEM
CHAPTER REVIEW SHEET 1

INSTRUCTIONS: Write the meaning of each word element in the space provided. Check your answers by referring to the word element review within the chapter.

WORD ELEMENT TO DEFINITION

WORD ELEMENT	DEFINITION
1. angi/o	
2. aneurysm/o	
3. arter/o	
4. arteri/o	
5. arteriol/o	
6. ather/o	
7. cardi/o	
8. coron/o	
9. ech/o	
10. electr/o	

Number Correct_____X 10 Points Per Correct Answer: Your Score_____%

CHAPTER 10: CARDIOVASCULAR SYSTEM CHAPTER REVIEW SHEET 2

INSTRUCTIONS: Write the appropriate word element for each definition given. Place your answer in the space provided. Check your answers by referring to the word element review within the chapter.

DEFINITION TO WORD ELEMENT

DEFINITION	WORD ELEMENT
1. vessel	
2. aneurysm	
3. artery	
4. artery (other than #3)	
5. arteriole	
6. fatty	
7. heart	
8. heart (other than #7)	
9. sound	
10. electrical	

Number Correct_____X 10 Points Per Correct Answer: Your Score_____%

CHAPTER 11: RESPIRATORY SYSTEM CHAPTER REVIEW SHEET 1

INSTRUCTIONS: Write the meaning of each word element in the space provided. Check your answers by referring to the word element review within the chapter.

WORD ELEMENT TO DEFINITION

WORD ELEMENT	DEFINITION
1. alveol/o	
2. bronch/o	
3. epiglott/o	
4. laryng/o	
5. nas/o, rhin/o	
6. orth/o	
7. pector/o	
8. pharyng/o	
9. phren/o	
10. pleur/o	
11. pne/o	
12. pneum/o	
13. pneumon/o	
14. pulmon/o	
15. rhin/o, nas/o	
16. sinus/o	
17. thorac/o	
18. trache/o	
19. scop/o	
20. bronchiol/o	

Number Correct_____X 05 Points Per Correct Answer: Your Score_____%

CHAPTER 11: RESPIRATORY SYSTEM
CHAPTER REVIEW SHEET 2

INSTRUCTIONS: Write the appropriate word element for each definition given. Place your answer in the space provided. Check your answers by referring to the word element review within the chapter.

DEFINITION TO WORD ELEMENT

DEFINITION	WORD ELEMENT
1. alveolus	
2. bronchus	
3. epiglottis	
4. larynx	
5. nose	
6. straight	
7. chest	
8. pharynx	
9. diaphragm	
10. pleura	
11. breathing	
12. lung, air	
13. lung, air (other than #12)	
14. lungs	
15. nose (other than #5)	
16. sinus	
17. chest (other than #7)	
18. trachea	
19. to view	
20. bronchiole	

Number Correct_____X 05 Points Per Correct Answer: Your Score_____%

CHAPTER 12: DIGESTIVE SYSTEM CHAPTER REVIEW SHEET 1

INSTRUCTIONS: Write the meaning of each word element in the space provided. Check your answers by referring to the word element review within the chapter.

WORD ELEMENT TO DEFINITION

WORD ELEMENT	DEFINITION
1. amyl/o	
2. appendic/o, append/o	
3. bil/i	
4. bucc/o	
5. cec/o	
6. cheil/o	
7. chol/e	
8. col/o	
9. colon/o	
10. dent/o	
11. cholecyst/o	
12. duoden/o	
13. -ectasia	
14. -emesis	
15. enter/o	
16. esophag/o	
17. gastr/o	
18. gingiv/o	
19. gloss/o	
20. gluc/o, glyc/o	

Number Correct_____X 05 Points Per Correct Answer: Your Score_____%

CHAPTER 12: DIGESTIVE SYSTEM
CHAPTER REVIEW SHEET 2

INSTRUCTIONS: Write the appropriate word element for each definition given. Place your answer in the space provided. Check your answers by referring to the word element review within the chapter.

DEFINITION TO WORD ELEMENT

DEFINITION	WORD ELEMENT
1. starch	
2. appendix	
3. bile	
4. cheek	
5. cecum	
6. lips	
7. bile (other than #3)	
8. colon	
9. colon (other than #8)	
10. tooth	
11. gallbladder	
12. duodenum	
13. stretching (suffix)	
14. to vomit (suffix)	
15. intestines	
16. esophagus	
17. stomach	
18. gums	
19. tongue	
20. sugar, sweetness	

Number Correct_____X 05 Points Per Correct Answer: Your Score_____%

CHAPTER 12: DIGESTIVE SYSTEM
CHAPTER REVIEW SHEET 3

INSTRUCTIONS: Write the meaning of each word element in the space provided. Check your answers by referring to the word element review within the chapter.

WORD ELEMENT TO DEFINITION

WORD ELEMENT	DEFINITION
1. hepat/o	
2. ile/o	
3. jejun/o	
4. lapar/o	
5. lingu/o	
6. lip/o	
7. lith/o	
8. -lysis	
9. mandibul/o	
10. odont/o, dent/o	
11. or/o	
12. rect/o	
13. peritone/o	
14. -pepsia	
15. sial/o	
16. sigmoid/o	
17. steat/o	
18. stomat/o	
19. -tresia	
20. -tripsy	

Number Correct_____X 05 Points Per Correct Answer: Your Score_____%

CHAPTER 12: DIGESTIVE SYSTEM
CHAPTER REVIEW SHEET 4

INSTRUCTIONS: Write the appropriate word element for each definition given. Place your answer in the space provided. Check your answers by referring to the word element review within the chapter.

DEFINITION TO WORD ELEMENT

DEFINITION	WORD ELEMENT
1. liver	
2. ileum	
3. jejunum	
4. abdominal wall	
5. tongue	
6. fat	
7. stone, calculus	
8. destruction (suffix)	
9. mandible	
10. teeth	
11. mouth	
12. rectum	
13. peritoneum	
14. state of digestion (suffix)	
15. saliva, salivary gland	
16. sigmoid colon	
17. fat (other than #6)	
18. mouth (other than #11)	
19. perforation (suffix)	
20. to crush (suffix)	

Number Correct_____X 05 Points Per Correct Answer: Your Score_____%

CHAPTER 13: ENDOCRINE SYSTEM
CHAPTER REVIEW SHEET 1

INSTRUCTIONS: Write the meaning of each word element in the space provided. Check your answers by referring to the word element review within the chapter.

WORD ELEMENT TO DEFINITION

WORD ELEMENT	DEFINITION
1. acr/o	
2. aden/o	
3. andr/o	
4. calc/o	
5. cortic/o	
6. crin/o, -crine	
7. dips/o, -dipsia	
8. kal/i	
9. lact/o	
10. myx/o	
11. natr/o	
12. oxy-	
13. pancreat/o	
14. somat/o	
15. thyr/o, thyroid/o	
16. thym/o	
17. toxic/o	
18. -tropin	
19. -uria	
20. gonad/o	

Number Correct_____X 05 Points Per Correct Answer: Your Score_____%

CHAPTER 13: ENDOCRINE SYSTEM CHAPTER REVIEW SHEET 2

INSTRUCTIONS: Write the appropriate word element for each definition given. Place your answer in the space provided. Check your answers by referring to the word element review within the chapter.

DEFINITION TO WORD ELEMENT

DEFINITION	WORD ELEMENT
1. extremities	
2. gland	
3. male	
4. calcium	
5. cortex	
6. secrete	
7. thirst	
8. potassium	
9. milk	
10. relating to mucus	
11. sodium	
12. sharp, quick (prefix)	
13. pancreas	
14. body	
15. thyroid gland	
16. thymus gland	
17. poisons	
18. stimulating effect of a hormone (suffix)	
19. urine condition (suffix)	
20. sex glands	

Number Correct_____X 05 Points Per Correct Answer: Your Score_____%

CHAPTER 14: SPECIAL SENSES
CHAPTER REVIEW SHEET 1

INSTRUCTIONS: Write the meaning of each word element in the space provided. Check your answers by referring to the word element review within the chapter.

WORD ELEMENT TO DEFINITION

WORD ELEMENT	DEFINITION
1. ambly/o	
2. aque/o	
3. blephar/o	
4. corne/o	
5. cor/o	
6. conjunctiv/o	
7. dacry/o	
8. es/o	
9. ex/o	
10. glauc/o	
11. ir/o	
12. irid/o	
13. kerat/o	
14. lacrim/o	
15. mi/o	
16. nas/o	
17. ocul/o	
18. ophthalm/o	
19. -opia	
20. -opsia	

Number Correct_____X 05 Points Per Correct Answer: Your Score_____%

CHAPTER 14: SPECIAL SENSES
CHAPTER REVIEW SHEET 2

INSTRUCTIONS: Write the appropriate word element for each definition given. Place your answer in the space provided. Check your answers by referring to the word element review within the chapter.

DEFINITION TO WORD ELEMENT

DEFINITION	WORD ELEMENT
1. dull	
2. watery	
3. eyelid	
4. cornea	
5. pupil	
6. conjunctiva	
7. tears	
8. within	
9. outward	
10. gray, silver	
11. iris	
12. iris (other than #11)	
13. cornea (other than #4)	
14. tears (other than #7)	
15. smaller	
16. nose	
17. eye	
18. eye (other than #17)	
19. vision (suffix)	
20. vision (suffix other than #19)	

Number Correct_____X 05 Points Per Correct Answer: Your Score_____%

CHAPTER 14: SPECIAL SENSES
CHAPTER REVIEW SHEET 3

INSTRUCTIONS: Write the meaning of each word element in the space provided. Check your answers by referring to the word element review within the chapter.

WORD ELEMENT TO DEFINITION

WORD ELEMENT	DEFINITION
1. phac/o, phak/o	
2. phot/o	
3. pupill/o, cor/o	
4. retin/o	
5. scler/o	
6. vitre/o	
7. xer/o	
8. acous/o	
9. audi/o	
10. labyrinth/o	
11. myring/o	
12. tympan/o	
13. ot/o	
14. scot/o	
15. palpebr/o, blephar/o	
16. -ptosis	
17. opt/o, optic/o	
18. extra-	
19. epi-	
20. hemi-	

Number Correct_____X 05 Points Per Correct Answer: Your Score_____%

CHAPTER 14: SPECIAL SENSES
CHAPTER REVIEW SHEET 4

INSTRUCTIONS: Write the appropriate word element for each definition given. Place your answer in the space provided. Check your answers by referring to the word element review within the chapter.

DEFINITION TO WORD ELEMENT

DEFINITION	WORD ELEMENT
1. lens	
2. light	
3. pupil	
4. retina	
5. hard	
6. glassy	
7. dry	
8. hearing	
9. hearing (other than #8)	
10. inner ear	
11. eardrum	
12. eardrum (other than #11)	
13. ear	
14. darkness	
15. eyelid	
16. drooping (suffix)	
17. eye, vision	
18. outside of (prefix)	
19. upon (prefix)	
20. half (prefix)	

Number Correct_____X 05 Points Per Correct Answer: Your Score_____%

CHAPTER 15: URINARY SYSTEM
CHAPTER REVIEW SHEET 1

INSTRUCTIONS: Write the meaning of each word element in the space provided. Check your answers by referring to the word element review within the chapter.

WORD ELEMENT TO DEFINITION

WORD ELEMENT	DEFINITION
1. albumin/o	
2. azot/o	
3. bacteri/o	
4. cali/o, calic/o	
5. cyst/o	
6. dips/o	
7. glomerul/o	
8. ket/o, keton/o	
9. meat/o	
10. noct/i	
11. nephr/o	
12. ren/o	
13. olig/o	
14. pyel/o	
15. py/o	
16. ureter/o	
17. urethr/o	
18. ur/o	
19. urin/o	
20. vesic/o	

Number Correct_____X 05 Points Per Correct Answer: Your Score_____%

CHAPTER 15: URINARY SYSTEM CHAPTER REVIEW SHEET 2

INSTRUCTIONS: Write the appropriate word element for each definition given. Place your answer in the space provided. Check your answers by referring to the word element review within the chapter.

DEFINITION TO WORD ELEMENT

DEFINITION	WORD ELEMENT
1. albumin	
2. nitrogen	
3. bacteria	
4. calyx, calyces	
5. urinary bladder	
6. thirst	
7. glomerulus	
8. ketone bodies	
9. meatus	
10. night	
11. kidney	
12. kidney (other than #11)	
13. scanty	
14. renal pelvis	
15. pus	
16. ureter	
17. urethra	
18. urine	
19. urine (other than #18)	
20. urinary bladder (other than #5)	

Number Correct______X 05 Points Per Correct Answer: Your Score______%

CHAPTER 16: MALE REPRODUCTIVE SYSTEM CHAPTER REVIEW SHEET 1

INSTRUCTIONS: Write the meaning of each word element in the space provided. Check your answers by referring to the word element review within the chapter.

WORD ELEMENT TO DEFINITION

WORD ELEMENT	DEFINITION
1. balan/o	
2. crypt/o	
3. epididym/o	
4. hydr/o	
5. orchi/o, orch/o, orchid/o	
6. semin/i	
7. sperm/o, spermat/o	
8. prostat/o	
9. vas/o	
10. zo/o	

Number Correct_____X 10 Points Per Correct Answer: Your Score_____%

CHAPTER 16: MALE REPRODUCTIVE SYSTEM CHAPTER REVIEW SHEET 2

INSTRUCTIONS: Write the appropriate word element for each definition given. Place your answer in the space provided. Check your answers by referring to the word element review within the chapter.

DEFINITION TO WORD ELEMENT

DEFINITION	WORD ELEMENT
1. glans penis	
2. hidden	
3. epididymis	
4. water	
5. testicle	
6. semen	
7. sperm	
8. prostate gland	
9. vessel	
10. animal (man)	

Number Correct_____X 10 Points Per Correct Answer: Your Score_____%

CHAPTER 17: FEMALE REPRODUCTIVE SYSTEM
CHAPTER REVIEW SHEET 1

INSTRUCTIONS: Write the meaning of each word element in the space provided. Check your answers by referring to the word element review within the chapter.

WORD ELEMENT TO DEFINITION

WORD ELEMENT	DEFINITION
1. -arche	
2. cervic/o	
3. colp/o	
4. gynec/o	
5. hyster/o	
6. mamm/o	
7. men/o	
8. metr/o, metri/o	
9. mast/o	
10. o/o	
11. oophor/o	
12. -rrhea	
13. salping/o	
14. vagin/o	
15. vulv/o	
16. uter/o	
17. ovari/o	
18. ov/o	
19. ante-	
20. dys-	

Number Correct_____X 05 Points Per Correct Answer: Your Score_____%

CHAPTER 17: FEMALE REPRODUCTIVE SYSTEM CHAPTER REVIEW SHEET 2

INSTRUCTIONS: Write the appropriate word element for each definition given. Place your answer in the space provided. Check your answers by referring to the word element review within the chapter.

DEFINITION TO WORD ELEMENT

DEFINITION	WORD ELEMENT
1. beginning (suffix)	
2. cervix	
3. vagina	
4. woman	
5. uterus	
6. breast	
7. menstruation	
8. uterus (other than #5)	
9. breast (other than #6)	
10. egg, ovum	
11. ovary	
12. discharge, flow (suffix)	
13. fallopian tubes	
14. vagina (other than #3)	
15. vulva	
16. uterus (other than #3 or #14)	
17. ovary (other than #11)	
18. egg, ovum (other than #10)	
19. before (prefix)	
20. bad, painful (prefix)	

Number Correct_____X 05 Points Per Correct Answer: Your Score_____%

CHAPTER 18: OBSTETRICS
CHAPTER REVIEW SHEET 1

INSTRUCTIONS: Write the meaning of each word element in the space provided. Check your answers by referring to the word element review within the chapter.

WORD ELEMENT TO DEFINITION

WORD ELEMENT	DEFINITION
1. amni/o	
2. ante-	
3. culd/o	
4. -cyesis	
5. episi/o	
6. fet/o	
7. -gravida	
8. hyper-	
9. lact/o	
10. multi-	
11. nat/o	
12. nulli-	
13. -para	
14. primi-	
15. obstetr/o	
16. perine/o	
17. salping/o	
18. -tocia	
19. vagin/o	
20. pelv/i	

Number Correct_____X 05 Points Per Correct Answer: Your Score_____%

CHAPTER 18: OBSTETRICS
CHAPTER REVIEW SHEET 2

INSTRUCTIONS: Write the appropriate word element for each definition given. Place your answer in the space provided. Check your answers by referring to the word element review within the chapter.

DEFINITION TO WORD ELEMENT

DEFINITION	WORD ELEMENT
1. amnion	
2. before (prefix)	
3. vagina	
4. pregnancy (suffix)	
5. vulva	
6. fetus	
7. pregnancy (suffix)	
8. excessive, high (prefix)	
9. milk	
10. many (prefix)	
11. birth	
12. none (prefix)	
13. to give birth (suffix)	
14. first (prefix)	
15. midwife	
16. perineum	
17. fallopian tube	
18. labor (suffix)	
19. vagina (other than #3)	
20. pelvis	

Number Correct_____X 05 Points Per Correct Answer: Your Score_____%

CHAPTER 19: CHILD HEALTH
CHAPTER REVIEW SHEET 1

INSTRUCTIONS: Write the meaning of each word element in the space provided. Check your answers by referring to the word element review within the chapter.

WORD ELEMENT TO DEFINITION

WORD ELEMENT	DEFINITION
1. cephal/o	
2. crypt/o	
3. hydr/o	
4. hypo-	
5. micr/o	
6. ne/o	
7. omphal/o	
8. pedi/a	
9. pyr/o	
10. tetr/a	

Number Correct_____X 10 Points Per Correct Answer: Your Score_____%

CHAPTER 19: CHILD HEALTH
CHAPTER REVIEW SHEET 2

INSTRUCTIONS: Write the appropriate word element for each definition given. Place your answer in the space provided. Check your answers by referring to the word element review within the chapter.

DEFINITION TO WORD ELEMENT

DEFINITION	WORD ELEMENT
1. head	
2. hidden	
3. water	
4. under (prefix)	
5. small	
6. new	
7. navel	
8. child	
9. heat, fire	
10. four	

Number Correct_____X 10 Points Per Correct Answer: Your Score_____%

CHAPTER 20: RADIOLOGY & DIAGNOSTIC IMAGING
CHAPTER REVIEW SHEET 1

INSTRUCTIONS: Write the meaning of each word element in the space provided. Check your answers by referring to the word element review within the chapter.

WORD ELEMENT TO DEFINITION

WORD ELEMENT	DEFINITION
1. angi/o	
2. anter/o	
3. arthr/o	
4. arteri/o	
5. cardi/o	
6. chol/e	
7. cine-	
8. ech/o	
9. fluor/o	
10. lymph/o	
11. myel/o	
12. poster/o	
13. pyel/o	
14. radi/o	
15. son/o	
16. tel/e	
17. tom/o	
18. ultra-	
19. ven/o	
20. xer/o	

Number Correct_____X 05 Points Per Correct Answer: Your Score_____%

CHAPTER 20: RADIOLOGY & DIAGNOSTIC IMAGING CHAPTER REVIEW SHEET 2

INSTRUCTIONS: Write the appropriate word element for each definition given. Place your answer in the space provided. Check your answers by referring to the word element review within the chapter.

DEFINITION TO WORD ELEMENT

DEFINITION	WORD ELEMENT
1. vessel	
2. front	
3. joint	
4. artery	
5. heart	
6. gall, bile	
7. pertaining to movement (prefix)	
8. sound	
9. luminous	
10. lymph	
11. bone marrow, spinal cord	
12. back	
13. renal pelvis	
14. radiation, x-ray	
15. sound (other than #8)	
16. distance	
17. to cut, section	
18. beyond (prefix)	
19. vein	
20. dry	

Number Correct_____X 05 Points Per Correct Answer: Your Score_____%

CHAPTER 21: ONCOLOGY
CHAPTER REVIEW SHEET 1

INSTRUCTIONS: Write the meaning of each word element in the space provided. Check your answers by referring to the word element review within the chapter.

WORD ELEMENT TO DEFINITION

WORD ELEMENT	DEFINITION
1. ana-	
2. -blast	
3. carcin/o	
4. chem/o	
5. meta-	
6. -oma	
7. onc/o	
8. sarc/o	
9. scirrh/o	
10. -plasia	

Number Correct_____X 10 Points Per Correct Answer: Your Score_____%

CHAPTER 21: ONCOLOGY
CHAPTER REVIEW SHEET 2

INSTRUCTIONS: Write the appropriate word element for each definition given. Place your answer in the space provided. Check your answers by referring to the word element review within the chapter.

DEFINITION TO WORD ELEMENT

DEFINITION	WORD ELEMENT
1. not, without (prefix)	
2. embryonic state of development (suffix)	
3. cancer	
4. pertaining to a chemical	
5. change (prefix)	
6. tumor (suffix)	
7. tumor (other than #6)	
8. of or related to flesh	
9. hard	
10. formation or development (suffix)	

Number Correct_____X 10 Points Per Correct Answer: Your Score_____%

CHAPTER 22: PHARMACOLOGY
CHAPTER REVIEW SHEET 1

INSTRUCTIONS: Write the meaning of each word element in the space provided. Check your answers by referring to the word element review within the chapter.

WORD ELEMENT TO DEFINITION

WORD ELEMENT	DEFINITION
1. alges/o	
2. anti-	
3. arrhythm/o	
4. bi/o	
5. bucc/o	
6. chem/o	
7. coagul/o	
8. ven/o	
9. esthesi/o	
10. fung/o	
11. gloss/o	
12. hyper-	
13. hypno-	
14. vagin/o	
15. rect/o	
16. -ist	
17. lingu/o	
18. -logy	
19. toxic/o	
20. or/o	

Number Correct_____X 05 Points Per Correct Answer: Your Score_____%

CHAPTER 22: PHARMACOLOGY
CHAPTER REVIEW SHEET 2

INSTRUCTIONS: Write the appropriate word element for each definition given. Place your answer in the space provided. Check your answers by referring to the word element review within the chapter.

DEFINITION TO WORD ELEMENT

DEFINITION	WORD ELEMENT
1. pain	
2. against (prefix)	
3. rhythm	
4. life	
5. cheek	
6. drug	
7. clotting	
8. vein	
9. feeling	
10. fungus	
11. tongue	
12. excessive, high (prefix)	
13. sleep (prefix)	
14. vagina	
15. rectum	
16. specialist (suffix)	
17. tongue (other than #11)	
18. the study of (suffix)	
19. poison	
20. mouth	

Number Correct_____X 05 Points Per Correct Answer: Your Score_____%

CHAPTER 23: MENTAL HEALTH
CHAPTER REVIEW SHEET 1

INSTRUCTIONS: Write the meaning of each word element in the space provided. Check your answers by referring to the word element review within the chapter.

WORD ELEMENT TO DEFINITION

WORD ELEMENT	DEFINITION
1. cata-	
2. hypn/o	
3. iatr/o	
4. -mania	
5. ment/o	
6. phil/o	
7. -phobia	
8. -phoria	
9. psych/o	
10. schiz/o	

Number Correct_____X 10 Points Per Correct Answer: Your Score_____%

CHAPTER 23: MENTAL HEALTH
CHAPTER REVIEW SHEET 2

INSTRUCTIONS: Write the appropriate word element for each definition given. Place your answer in the space provided. Check your answers by referring to the word element review within the chapter.

DEFINITION TO WORD ELEMENT

DEFINITION	WORD ELEMENT
1. down, under, against, lower (prefix)	
2. sleep	
3. pertaining to a physician or treatment	
4. madness (suffix)	
5. mind	
6. having a love for or a strong attraction to	
7. abnormal fear (suffix)	
8. emotional state (suffix)	
9. mind (other than #5)	
10. split, divided	

Number Correct_____X 10 Points Per Correct Answer: Your Score_____%

CHAPTER EXAMS

Included in this section are chapter exams for Chapters 2 through 23. Each exam consists of 50 questions: 20 multiple choice, 15 matching, and 15 completion questions.

The instructor will note that examples are given for the first ten questions of the exam in Chapter 2. The examples give a definition of a sample word with meaning of the prefix enclosed in quotation marks. This format is designed to help the learner solidify the meaning of the prefix in the early chapters of the text. An illustration is shown below.

3. A prefix that means **toward, increase** (as in movement "toward" the midline of the body) is
   a. a-　　　　c. auto-
   b. ad-　　　　d. bi-
   Answer: ad-

If the instructor does not wish to use this format, the example can easily be eliminated from the sample test and the learner can be tested on the definition alone, without an example.

For the exam in Chapter 3, most of the multiple choice questions ask the learner to define the given suffix or to identify the suffix based upon the given definition. When a medical term is used in the question, the part that relates directly to the suffix will be in quotes (" ") since this is still new to the learner. An illustration is shown below.

9. The word which means **surgical removal of the appendix** is
   a. appendices　　　　c. appendectomy
   b. appendiceal　　　　d. appendicitis
   Answer: appendectomy

Rationale: This type of question teaches the learner to see the word element as it appears in the word, locate the suffix, and define it.

For Chapters 5 through 23, alternate completion questions emphasizing word elements and abbreviations have been added. Included with each of these exams is an additional set of completion questions that concentrate on word elements and abbreviations, numbered 36 through 50 (answers included with answer key). These questions can be substituted for the completion questions in the exam if the instructor prefers, particularly if this is the only text that will be used to teach medical terminology.

EXTRA CREDIT: On occasion, the instructor may choose to use the alternate completion questions as extra credit questions, selecting eight of the completion questions and granting 1/4 point for each correct answer, for a total of two bonus points on the exam.

CHAPTER 2 PREFIXES
CHAPTER EXAM

MULTIPLE CHOICE

INSTRUCTIONS: The following questions or incomplete statements are followed by four answers or completions. Read each question carefully and select the most appropriate response.

1. A prefix that means **without, away from** (as in "without" breathing) is
   a. a-
   b. ad-
   c. auto-
   d. bi-
2. A prefix that means **from, away from** (as in wandering "away from") is
   a. ab-
   b. alb-
   c. an-
   d. ante-
3. A prefix that means **toward, increase** (as in movement "toward" the midline of the body) is
   a. a-
   b. ad-
   c. auto-
   d. bi-
4. A prefix that means **white** (as in abnormally "white" skin) is
   a. bio-
   b. auto-
   c. alb-
   d. rube-
5. A prefix that means **both, both sides** (as in able to use "both" hands well) is
   a. a-
   b. ad-
   c. ante-
   d. ambi-
6. A prefix that means **before, in front of** (as in the space "in front of" the elbow) is
   a. ambi-
   b. ante-
   c. auto-
   d. brady-
7. A prefix that means **against** (as in a substance that works "against" the action of poison) is
   a. circum-
   b. bi-
   c. anti-
   d. ante-
8. A prefix that means **self** (as in a graft of skin transferred from one part of "one's" body to another part) is
   a. auto-
   b. bi-
   c. pseudo-
   d. ambi-
9. A prefix that means **two, double** (as in having "two" cusps or points) is
   a. auto-
   b. bi-
   c. pseudo-
   d. mono-
10. A prefix that means **slow** (as in "slow" heart beat) is
    a. circum-
    b. ambi-
    c. auto-
    d. brady-
11. The prefix **circum-** means
    a. white
    b. around
    c. slow
    d. two, double
12. The prefix **con-** means
    a. together, with
    b. within
    c. likeness, same
    d. excessive

13. The prefix **dis-** means
    a. bad, difficult
    b. outside
    c. free of, to undo
    d. outside of, beyond

14. The prefix **dys-** means
    a. bad, difficult
    b. outside
    c. free of, to undo
    d. outside of, beyond

15. The prefix **ecto-** means
    a. good, normal
    b. outside
    c. within
    d. free of, to undo

16. The prefix **endo-** means
    a. good, normal
    b. outside
    c. within
    d. free of, to undo

17. The prefix **epi-** means
    a. half
    b. same
    c. outside
    d. upon, over

18. The prefix **eu-** means
    a. bad, difficult
    b. good, normal
    c. likeness, same
    d. excessive

19. The prefix **extra-** means
    a. outside of, beyond
    b. half
    c. away from
    d. upon, over

20. The prefix **homo-** means
    a. half
    b. different
    c. water
    d. same

MATCHING

INSTRUCTIONS: Match the prefix on the left with the correct definition on the right. Enter your selection in the space provided.

_____ 21. hydro-	a. beneath, under
_____ 22. hyper-	b. water
_____ 23. meta-	c. change, after
_____ 24. idio-	d. excessive
_____ 25. infra-	e. individual

_____ 26. inter-	a. one
_____ 27. juxta-	b. between
_____ 28. hypo-	c. one-thousandth
_____ 29. milli-	d. less than, under
_____ 30. mono-	e. near, beside

_____ 31. multi-	a. all
_____ 32. non-	b. many
_____ 33. pan-	c. near, beside
_____ 34. para-	d. not
_____ 35. per-	e. through

COMPLETION

INSTRUCTIONS: Read each statement carefully and complete the statement with the most appropriate response. Enter your answer in the space provided.

36. The prefix **poly-** means ____________________

37. The prefix **post-** means ____________________

38. The prefix **pre-** means ____________________

39. The prefix **primi-** means ____________________

40. The prefix **pseudo-** means ____________________

41. The prefix **retro-** means ____________________

42. The prefix **sub-** means ____________________

43. The prefix **supra-** means ____________________

44. The prefix that means **joined, together** is ____________________

45. The prefix that means **rapid** is ____________________

46. The prefix that means **across, through** is ____________________

47. The prefix that means **three** is ____________________

48. The prefix that means **one** is ____________________

49. The prefix that means **dry** is ____________________

50. The prefix that means **around** is ____________________

CHAPTER 3 SUFFIXES CHAPTER EXAM

MULTIPLE CHOICE

INSTRUCTIONS: The following questions or incomplete statements are followed by four answers or completions. Read each question carefully and select the most appropriate response.

1. A suffix that means **toward** is
   a. -ac
   b. -ad
   c. -ate
   d. -al

2. The suffix **-algesia** means
   a. sensitivity to pain
   b. pain
   c. herniation
   d. movement toward

3. The suffix **-algia** means
   a. sensitivity to pain
   b. pain
   c. herniation
   d. movement toward

4. The suffix that refers to **a surgical puncture** is
   a. -ectomy
   b. -otomy
   c. -centesis
   d. -ostomy

5. When building a word that refers to **cells**, you would use the suffix
   a. -cyst
   b. -cide
   c. -desis
   d. -cyte

6. The suffix **-dynia** means
   a. to kill, to destroy
   b. pain
   c. binding or fusion
   d. condition of

7. The suffix **-ectasia** means
   a. crushing or breaking up
   b. stretching or dilatation
   c. blood condition
   d. generating; formation

8. When using the suffix **-cide**, you know that the word will refer to a substance that
   a. kills or destroys
   b. generates or forms
   c. binds
   d. stretches or dilates

9. The word that means **surgical removal of the appendix** is
   a. appendices
   b. appendiceal
   c. appendectomy
   d. appendicitis

10. The suffix that refers to **a blood condition** is
    a. -emia
    b. -esis
    c. -lysis
    d. -cyte

11. **One who takes and processes x-rays** is known as a
    a. radiologist
    b. radiocist
    c. radiatrician
    d. radiographer

12. The suffix **-genesis** means
    a. pertaining to
    b. generating; formation
    c. binding or fusion
    d. condition

13. A **record or picture of the heart** is known as a
    a. cardiography
    b. cardiograph
    c. cardiogram
    d. cardiocentesis

14. An **instrument used to record the electrical activity of the heart** is known as a
    a. electrocardiography
    b. electrocardiograph
    c. electrocardiogram
    d. electrocardiocentesis

15. The **process of recording the electrical activity of the heart** is known as a
    a. cardiography
    b. cardiograph
    c. cardiogram
    d. cardiocentesis

16. The suffix that refers to **a specialist in a field of study** is
    a. -ical
    b. -ile
    c. -logy
    d. -iatrist

17. The suffix that refers to **a process or action** is
    a. -ion
    b. -ile
    c. -ical
    d. -ia

18. Identify the suffixes that mean **pertaining to**
    1. -ic
    2. -ac
    3. -al
    4. -cele
    5. -ar

    a. 1, 2, 3, 4
    b. 1, 2, 4, 5
    c. 1, 2, 3, 5
    d. 1, 2, 3, 4, 5

19. Identify the suffixes that mean **condition**
    1. -ia
    2. -ic
    3. -ism
    4. -osis
    5. -y

    a. 1, 3, 4
    b. 2, 3, 4
    c. 3, 4, 5
    d. 1, 3, 5

20. The word that means **inflammation of the appendix** is
    a. appendices
    b. appendiceal
    c. appendectomy
    d. appendicitis

MATCHING

INSTRUCTIONS: Match the suffix on the left with the correct definition on the right. Enter your selection in the space provided.

_____ 21. -lepsy	a. one who specializes in the study of
_____ 22. -lith	b. seizure
_____ 23. -lithiasis	c. stone
_____ 24. -logy	d. the study of
_____ 25. -logist	e. presence or formation of stones
_____ 26. -lysis	a. enlargement
_____ 27. -mania	b. the process of measuring
_____ 28. -megaly	c. destruction or detachment
_____ 29. -meter	d. madness
_____ 30. -metry	e. an instrument used to measure
_____ 31. -oid	a. condition
_____ 32. -ole	b. resembling
_____ 33. -oma	c. tumor
_____ 34. -opia	d. small or little
_____ 35. -osis	e. visual condition

COMPLETION

INSTRUCTIONS: Read each statement carefully and complete the statement with the most appropriate response. Enter your answer in the space provided.

36. The suffix **-pathy** means ______________________________

37. The suffix **-penia** means ______________________________

38. The suffix **-pexy** means ______________________________

39. The suffix **-philia** means ______________________________

40. The suffix **-phobia** means ______________________________

41. The suffix **-plasty** means ______________________________

42. The suffix **-plegia** means ______________________________

43. The suffix that means **breathing** is ______________________________

44. The suffix that means **prolapse** is ______________________________

45. The suffix that means **suturing** is ______________________________

46. The suffix that means **drainage** is ______________________________

47. The suffix that means **rupture** is ______________________________

48. The suffix that means **incision into** is ______________________________

49. The suffix that means **creating a new opening** is ______________________________

50. The suffix that means **surgical crushing** is ______________________________

CHAPTER 4 WHOLE BODY TERMS CHAPTER EXAM

MULTIPLE CHOICE

INSTRUCTIONS: The following questions or incomplete statements are followed by four answers or completions. Read each question carefully and select the most appropriate response.

1. A change in the structure and orientation of cells, characterized by a loss of differentiation and reversion to a more primitive form is known as
   a. dysplasia — c. hypoplasia
   b. anaplasia — d. aplasia

2. A developmental failure resulting in the absence of any organ or tissue is known as
   a. dysplasia — c. hypoplasia
   b. anaplasia — d. aplasia

3. Any abnormal development of tissues or organs is known as
   a. dysplasia — c. hypoplasia
   b. anaplasia — d. aplasia

4. The body cavity containing the liver, gallbladder, spleen, stomach, pancreas, intestines, and kidneys is the
   a. thoracic cavity — c. pelvic cavity
   b. abdominal cavity — d. cranial cavity

5. The position in which the person is standing with the arms at the sides and the palms turned forward, with the individual's head and feet pointing forward is known as
   a. anteroposterior position — c. anatomical position
   b. posteroanterior position — d. cephalocaudal position

6. The term that means pertaining to the tail is
   a. cephalic — c. lateral
   b. caudal — d. dorsal

7. The semipermeable barrier that is the outer covering of a cell is the
   a. cytoplasm — c. mitochondria
   b. nucleus — d. cell membrane

8. Tissue that supports and binds other body tissue and parts is known as
   a. connective tissue — c. striated muscle
   b. epithelial tissue — d. subcutaneous tissue

9. The segments of chromosomes that transmit hereditary characteristics are known as
   a. genes — c. nephrons
   b. neurons — d. cytoplasm

10. A medical scientist who specializes in the study of tissues is called a
    a. tissologist — c. neurologist
    b. histologist — d. dermatologist

11. Incomplete development or underdevelopment of an organ or tissue is called
    a. hyperplasia — c. hypoplasia
    b. neoplasia — d. aplasia

12. The term that means pertaining to the internal organs is
    a. ventral — c. caudal
    b. dorsal — d. visceral

13. A point on the right side of the abdomen about two thirds of the distance between the umbilicus and the anterior bony prominence of the hip is known as ________. Tenderness over this point might make the physician suspect appendicitis.
    a. McBurney's Point
    b. Monroe's Point
    c. Point of Pain
    d. Anterumbilical Point

14. The imaginary line that is created when the body is divided into equal right and left halves is known as the
    a. saggital plane
    b. midline of the body
    c. transverse line of the body
    d. mediolateral plane

15. The body cavity that contains the lungs, heart, aorta, esophagus, and the trachea is known as the
    a. pelvic cavity
    b. cranial cavity
    c. thoracic cavity
    d. abdominal cavity

16. The medical term for the navel or "belly button" is
    a. umbilicus
    b. ilium
    c. cecum
    d. navocele

17. The central controlling body within a living cell that is enclosed within the cell membrane is the
    a. cytoplasm
    b. nucleus
    c. mitochondria
    d. riboplasm

18. A specific, serous membrane that covers the entire abdominal wall of the body is the
    a. perineum
    b. parietal pleura
    c. cytoplasm
    d. peritoneum

19. Tissue that transmits impulses throughout the body, thereby activating, coordinating, and controlling the many functions of the body is
    a. nervous tissue
    b. muscle tissue
    c. epithelial tissue
    d. skeletal tissue

20. Another name for smooth muscle, that is found in the walls of the hollow internal organs of the body such as the stomach and intestines is
    a. skeletal muscle
    b. epithelial muscle
    c. visceral muscle
    d. cardiac muscle

MATCHING

INSTRUCTIONS: Match the term on the left with the correct definition on the right. Enter your selection in the space provided.

_____ 21. proximal	a. lying horizontally on the back, face up
_____ 22. prone	b. toward or nearest to the trunk of the body or point of origin
_____ 23. supine	c. lying face down on the abdomen
_____ 24. superficial	d. above or upward toward the head
_____ 25. superior	e. near the surface

_____ 26. mediolateral	a. pertaining to the back
_____ 27. ventral	b. below or downward toward the tail or feet
_____ 28. lateral	c. toward the side of the body
_____ 29. inferior	d. pertaining to the middle and side of a structure
_____ 30. dorsal	e. pertaining to the front; belly-side

_____	31. caudal	a. a movement that allows the palms to turn upward or forward
_____	32. anterior	b. pertaining to the back of the body
_____	33. medial	c. pertaining to the tail
_____	34. supination	d. pertaining to the front of the body or toward the belly of the body
_____	35. posterior	e. toward the midline of the body

COMPLETION

INSTRUCTIONS: Read each statement carefully and complete the statement with the most appropriate response. Enter your answer in the space provided.

36. The combining form **anter/o** means ____________________

37. The combining form **cyt/o** means ____________________

38. The combining form **hist/o** means ____________________

39. The combining form **inguin/o** means ____________________

40. The combining form **later/o** means ____________________

41. The combining form **poster/o** means ____________________

42. The combining form **proxim/o** means ____________________

43. The combining form **ventr/o** means ____________________

44. The prefix that means **not, without** is ____________________

45. The combining form that means **neck** is ____________________

46. The prefix that means **below, under** is ____________________

47. The prefix that means **between** is ____________________

48. The combining form that means **middle** is ____________________

49. The combining form that means **navel** is ____________________

50. The prefix that means **upon** is ____________________

CHAPTER 5 INTEGUMENTARY SYSTEM CHAPTER EXAM

MULTIPLE CHOICE

INSTRUCTIONS: The following questions or incomplete statements are followed by four answers or completions. Read each question carefully and select the most appropriate response.

1. A common inflammatory disorder seen on the face, chest, back, and neck that appears as papules, pustules, and comedos is
   a. acne vulgaris
   b. albinism
   c. eczema
   d. impetigo

2. A condition characterized by absence of pigment in the skin, hair, and eyes is known as
   a. acne vulgaris
   b. albinism
   c. eczema
   d. leukoplakia

3. Second degree or partial thickness burns
   1. exhibit a blistering pink to red color with some swelling.
   2. involve the epidermis and upper layer of the dermis.
   3. are very sensitive and painful.
   4. heal in approximately two weeks without a scar if no wound infection or trauma occur during the healing process.
   5. exhibit no blistering.

   a. 2, 3, 5
   b. 2, 3, 4
   c. 2, 3, 4, 5
   d. 1, 2, 3, 4

4. The most common malignant tumor of the epithelial tissue that occurs most often on areas of the skin exposed to the sun is
   a. malignant melanoma
   b. astrocytoma
   c. basal cell carcinoma
   d. adenocarcinoma

5. Examples of exanthematous viral diseases include which of the following?
   1. Rubella (German measles)
   2. Roseola infantum
   3. Rubeola (measles)
   4. Erythema infectiosum (fifth disease)

   a. 1, 2
   b. 2, 3
   c. 1, 2, 3
   d. 1, 2, 3, 4

6. Tissue death due to the loss of adequate blood supply, invasion of bacteria, and subsequent decay, producing a very offensive foul odor is known as
   a. gangrene
   b. impetigo
   c. leukoplakia
   d. cellulitis

7. An acute viral infection characterized by painful, vesicular eruptions on the skin following along the nerve pathways of underlying spinal or cranial nerves is known as
   a. Kaposi's sarcoma
   b. shingles (herpes zoster)
   c. herpes simplex
   d. genital herpes

8. A highly contagious superficial skin infection characterized by serous vesicles and pustules that form crusts is known as
   a. leukoplakia c. impetigo
   b. eczema d. shingles
9. A rare, malignant lesion, associated with AIDS, that begins as a soft purple-brown nodule or plaque on the feet and gradually spreads throughout the skin is known as
   a. Kaposi's sarcoma c. basal cell carcinoma
   b. shingles d. lymphoma
10. Overstretching of the elastic fibers of the dermis, due to obesity or pregnancy, results in linear tears in the dermis that are known as
    a. stria c. petechia
    b. white patches d. elastins
11. White, hard, thickened patches firmly attached to the mucous membrane in areas such as the mouth, vulva, or penis are known as
    a. plaque c. leukoplakia
    b. erythremia d. ulcers
12. A common noninfectious chronic disorder of the skin manifested by silvery white scales over round, raised, reddened plaques, occurring largely on the scalp, ears, extensor surfaces of the extremities, and bony prominences is known as
    a. impetigo c. eczema
    b. scabies d. psoriasis
13. A highly contagious parasitic infestation caused by the "human itch mite" causing a rash, pruritus, and a feeling of something crawling on the skin is known as
    a. shingles c. eczema
    b. scabies d. impetigo
14. A chronic multisystem inflammatory disease characterized by lesions of the nervous system and skin, renal problems, vasculitis, and a red "butterfly rash" on the nose and face is
    a. systemic lupus erythematosus c. myasthenia gravis
    b. leukoplakia d. roseola
15. Ringworm of the scalp is known as
    a. tinea pedis c. tinea cruris
    b. tinea capitis d. tinea corpis
16. Examples of various procedures used to identify specific allergens in an individual by exposing the person to a very small quantity of the allergen include
    1. intradermal injections
    2. patch testing
    3. scratch tests
    4. intravenous injections

    a. 1, 2, 3 c. 1, 3, 4
    b. 2, 3, 4 d. 1, 3, 4
17. A noninvasive treatment for non-melanoma skin cancer using liquid nitrogen that freezes the tissue is known as
    a. electrocauterization c. electrodessication
    b. cryosurgery d. dermabrasion

18. Removal of debris, foreign objects, and damaged or necrotic tissue from a wound in order to prevent infection and promote healing is known as
    a. electrocauterization
    b. aseptic cleansing
    c. denecrosing
    d. debridement

19. Aspiration of fat through a suction cannula or curette to alter the body contours is known as
    a. liposuction
    b. aspiration biopsy
    c. atherectomy
    d. curettage

20. The removal of a small piece of tissue from skin lesions for the purpose of examining it under a microscope to confirm or establish a diagnosis.
    a. dermectomy
    b. debridement
    c. exfoliative cytology
    d. skin biopsy

MATCHING

INSTRUCTIONS: Match the term on the left with the correct definition on the right. Enter your selection in the space provided.

_____ 21. abscess
_____ 22. abrasion
_____ 23. blister
_____ 24. bruise
_____ 25. cerumen

a. ear wax
b. localized collection of pus in any part of the body
c. bluish-black discoloration of an area of the skin or mucous membrane
d. vesicle
e. scraping or rubbing away of skin or mucous membrane as a result of friction to the area

_____ 26. contusion
_____ 27. fissure
_____ 28. macule
_____ 29. papule
_____ 30. petechia

a. a crack-like sore or groove in the skin or mucous membrane
b. an injury to a part of the body without a break in the skin
c. small, pinpoint hemorrhages of the skin
d. a small, flat, discoloration that is neither raised nor depressed
e. a small, solid, circumscribed elevation on the skin

_____ 31. polyp
_____ 32. scales
_____ 33. skin tags
_____ 34. vesicle
_____ 35. wheal

a. a small stalk-like growth that protrudes upward or outward from a mucous membrane
b. small brownish-colored or flesh-colored outgrowths of the skin, occurring frequently on the neck
c. a circumscribed, slightly elevated lesion of the skin that is paler in the center than its surrounding edges
d. thin flakes of hardened epithelium that are shed from the epidermis
e. a small, thin-walled skin lesion containing clear fluid

COMPLETION

INSTRUCTIONS: Read each statement carefully and complete the statement with the most appropriate response. Enter your answer in the space provided.

36. A circumscribed, open sore or lesion of the skin that is accompanied by inflammation is known as a(n) ____________

37. The clear watery fluid produced by sweat glands is called ____________

38. Another name for a sudoriferous gland is ____________

39. The fatty layer of tissue located beneath the dermis is known as the ____________

40. Linear tears in the dermis due to overstretching from rapid growth are called ____________

41. The oily secretion of the sebaceous glands is ____________

42. Another name for itching is ____________

43. Infestation with lice is known as ____________

44. The crescent-shaped, pale area at the base of the fingernail or toenail is known as the ____________

45. A tear in the skin is called a ____________

46. The tiny tube within the dermis that contains the root of a hair shaft is the ____________

47. The outermost layer of the skin is the ____________

48. A physician who specializes in the treatment of diseases and disorders of the skin is known as a ____________

49. Another name for the dermis, the layer of skin just under the epidermis, is the ____________

50. A diffused, acute infection of the skin and subcutaneous tissue, characterized by localized heat, deep redness, pain, and swelling is known as ____________

CHAPTER 5 ALTERNATE COMPLETION QUESTIONS
Emphasizing Word Elements and Abbreviations

(Can be substituted for Completion Questions 36-50)

COMPLETION

INSTRUCTIONS: Read each statement carefully and complete the statement with the most appropriate response. Enter your answer in the space provided.

36. The combining form **cutane/o** means ____________________

37. The combining form **derm/o** means ____________________

38. The combining form **kerat/o** means ____________________

39. The combining form **lip/o** means ____________________

40. The combining form **melan/o** means ____________________

41. The combining form **myc/o** means ____________________

42. The combining form **onych/o** means ____________________

43. The combining form that means **fish** is ____________________

44. The combining form for **yellow** is ____________________

45. The combining form for **white** is ____________________

46. The abbreviation for **biopsy** is ____________________

47. The abbreviation for **intradermal** is ____________________

48. The abbreviation for **incision and drainage** is ____________________

49. The abbreviation for **purified protein derivative** is ____________________

50. The abbreviation for **ointment** is ____________________

CHAPTER 6 SKELETAL SYSTEM CHAPTER EXAM

MULTIPLE CHOICE

INSTRUCTIONS: The following questions or incomplete statements are followed by four answers or completions. Read each question carefully and select the most appropriate response.

1. The rounded depression, or socket, in the pelvic bone where the thigh bone joins with the pelvis is called the
   a. acetabulum　　c. bursae
   b. acromion　　d. condyle

2. A joint is called a (an)
   a. acromion　　c. epiphysis
   b. articulation　　d. fascia

3. The connective tissue binding muscles to bones is called
   a. tendons　　c. ligaments
   b. cartilage　　d. fascia

4. Freely movable joints are called
   a. synovial joints　　c. synoveal joints
   b. sinovial joints　　d. synoveol joints

5. The connective tissue that binds bones to bones is
   a. tendons　　c. ligaments
   b. cartilage　　d. fascia

6. The process of bone formation is
   a. mastoid process　　c. synarthrosis
   b. sequestration　　d. ossification

7. An air cavity within bone is called a
   a. sinus　　c. spur
   b. vertebral arch　　d. sulcus

8. The muscles attached to bones are called voluntary or striated muscles. Another name for a striated muscle is
   a. skeletal　　c. visceral
   b. smooth　　d. synovial

9. Another name for involuntary muscles in the viscera and blood vessels is
   a. skeletal　　c. striated
   b. smooth　　d. synovial

10. The lower, narrow portion of the breast bone is the
    a. fontanelle　　c. tuberosity
    b. xiphoid process　　d. sarcolemma

11. The large process below the neck of the femur for muscle attachments is the
    a. trochanter　　c. olecranon
    b. tubercle　　d. sulcus

12. The first seven pairs of ribs, that articulate with the sternum, are known as the
    a. xiphoid process　　c. true ribs
    b. false ribs　　d. floating ribs

13. The superior part of the ilium is known as the
    a. iliac crust
    b. iliac spine
    c. iliac region
    d. iliac crest

14. The membrane surrounding the bones is the
    a. periosteum
    b. osteoclast
    c. medullary cavity
    d. perineum

15. A condition that occurs mainly in the hips and legs of older individuals and is characterized by chronic inflammation of bones and joints due to degenerative changes in cartilage is
    a. rheumatoid arthritis
    b. spondylosis
    c. osteoarthritis
    d. systemic lupus erythematosus

16. Swollen, painful joints accompanied by fever are symptoms of a chronic disease that affects women more commonly than men. This chronic disease, affecting the small joints of the hands and feet at first, is known as
    a. gout
    b. rheumatoid arthritis
    c. osteoma
    d. spondylosis

17. A group of inherited diseases characterized by progressive weakness and degeneration of muscle fibers without involvement of the nervous system is termed
    a. muscular dystrophy
    b. polymyalgia rheumatica
    c. bursitis
    d. multiple sclerosis

18. The cranial bone that composes the forehead and part of the eye socket is the
    a. parietal bone
    b. occipital bone
    c. frontal bone
    d. temporal bone

19. The cranial bone that composes the back and base of the skull is the
    a. parietal bone
    b. occipital bone
    c. frontal bone
    d. temporal bone

20. The mandible is commonly called the
    a. tear duct
    b. cheek
    c. nose
    d. jaw

MATCHING

INSTRUCTIONS: Match the term on the left with the correct definition on the right. Enter your selection in the space provided.

_____ 21. sternum	a. the knee cap
_____ 22. tarsals	b. the upper arm bone
_____ 23. ischium	c. the breastbone
_____ 24. humerus	d. the ankle bones
_____ 25. patella	e. the posterior part of the pelvic bone

_____ 26. phalanges	a. the medial lower arm bone, pinkie side
_____ 27. ilium	b. the shoulder bone
_____ 28. ulna	c. the wrist bones
_____ 29. carpals	d. the finger or toe bones
_____ 30. scapula	e. the uppermost part of the pelvic bone

_____	31. tibia	a. the smaller of the two bones in the lower leg
_____	32. femur	b. the lateral lower arm bone
_____	33. fibula	c. the larger of the two bones in the lower leg
_____	34. clavicle	d. the thigh bone
_____	35. radius	e. the collar bone

COMPLETION

INSTRUCTIONS: Read each statement carefully and complete the statement with the most appropriate response. Enter your answer in the space provided.

36. The junction line where two bones form a joint that does not permit any movement is known as a ____________________

37. Each end of a long bone is known as a(n) ____________________

38. Inflammation of bone marrow due to bacterial invasion of bone is known as ____________________

39. The cranial bones, composed of the lower sides and base of the cranium, are the ____________________

40. The thin, small bones, located at the corner of each eye, that contain fossa for the tear gland and canals for the passage of the tear duct are the ____________________

41. Rib pairs 8-10 connect to the vertebrae in the back but not to the sternum in the front because they join the 7th rib in the front. These rib pairs are known as ____________________

42. The spaces between the ribs are called ____________________

43. The process of bone formation is called ____________________

44. Mature bone cells are called ____________________

45. A condition/disease in which the bones become abnormally soft, due to a deficiency of calcium and phosphorus in the blood is known as ____________________

46. A fracture that occurs when a direct force breaks the bone, forcing the broken end of the smaller bone into the broken end of the larger bone is what type of fracture? ____________________

47. A fracture that occurs at the lower end of the radius, within one inch of connecting with the wrist bones is known as what type of fracture? ____________________

48. A hairline fracture is also known as what type of fracture? ____________________

49. When a bone is weakened by a pre-existing disease and breaks in response to a force that would not cause a normal bone to break, it is called a ____________________ fracture.

50. Realigning a broken bone under direct observation during surgery is called a(n) ____________________

CHAPTER 6 ALTERNATE COMPLETION QUESTIONS
Emphasizing Word Elements and Abbreviations

(Can be substituted for Completion Questions 36-50)

COMPLETION

INSTRUCTIONS: Read each statement carefully and complete the statement with the most appropriate response. Enter your answer in the space provided.

36. The combining form **oste/o** means ____________________________________

37. The combining form **vertebr/o** means ____________________________________

38. The combining form **kyph/o** means ____________________________________

39. The combining form **lord/o** means ____________________________________

40. The combining form **scoli/o** means ____________________________________

41. The combining form **cost/o** refers to the ____________________________________

42. The medical word that means **inflammation of bone and bone marrow** is ____________________

43. The **outward extension of the scapula that forms the point of the shoulder** is the ________________

44. A **closed fracture** is one that has ____________________________________

45. A **greenstick fracture** is one that has ____________________________________

46. The abbreviation for **dual-energy x-ray absorptiometry** is __________________________

47. The abbreviation for **fracture** is ____________________________________

48. When referring to the **second lumbar vertebra**, the abbreviation would be written as ________________

49. The abbreviation for **total knee replacement** is ____________________________________

50. The abbreviation for **temporomandibular joint** is ____________________________________

CHAPTER 7 MUSCLES AND JOINTS CHAPTER EXAM

MULTIPLE CHOICE

INSTRUCTIONS: The following questions or incomplete statements are followed by four answers or completions. Read each question carefully and select the most appropriate response.

1. A genetically transmitted disorder that is characterized by progressive weakness and muscle fiber degeneration without evidence of nerve involvement or degeneration of nerve tissue is known as
   a. muscular dystrophy
   b. multiple sclerosis
   c. scleroderma
   d. muscle strain
2. An injury to the body of the muscle or attachment of the tendon, as a result of overstretching, overextension, or misuse; ie, a "muscle pull", is also called a
   a. torn ligament
   b. subluxation
   c. myocele
   d. muscle strain
3. The process of recording the strength of the contraction of a muscle when it is stimulated by an electrical current is known as
   a. electroencephalography
   b. electromyography
   c. myelography
   d. electromycography
4. Inflammation of the joints is known as
   a. spondylosis
   b. arthritis
   c. spondylitis
   d. tendonitis
5. An abnormal enlargement of the joint at the base of the great toe is called a
   a. ganglion
   b. cyst
   c. bursa
   d. bunion
6. A cystic tumor developing on a tendon, that sometimes occurs on the back of the wrist, is known as a
   a. ganglion
   b. cyst
   c. bursa
   d. bunion
7. A form of acute arthritis that is characterized by inflammation of the first metatarsal joint of the great toe is known as
   a. polyarthritis
   b. osteoarthritis
   c. gout
   d. rheumatoid arthritis
8. An acute, recurrent inflammatory infection, transmitted through the bite of an infected deer tick is known as
   a. Lyme disease
   b. Rocky Mountain Spotted Fever
   c. Kaposi's sarcoma
   d. Huntington's chorea
9. Symptoms of the infection identified in Question 8 (above) include which of the following?
   1. a circular rash (a red, itchy rash with a circular center)
   2. influenza-like symptoms: weakness, chills, fever, headaches, and muscle or joint pain
   3. a purplish, spotted rash
   4. pruritus

   a. 1, 2
   b. 1, 4
   c. 2, 3
   d. 3, 4

10. The most common form of arthritis, due to wear and tear on the joints, especially the weight-bearing joints such as the hips and knees, is
    a. rheumatoid arthritis
    b. osteoarthritis
    c. gout
    d. polyarthritis

11. A chronic type of arthritis that affects multiple joints of the body, mainly the small peripheral joints, as in those of the hands and feet is known as
    a. rheumatoid arthritis
    b. osteoarthritis
    c. gout
    d. polyarthritis

12. The surgical puncture of a joint with a needle, for the purpose of withdrawing fluid for analysis is known as an
    a. arthrocentesis
    b. arthroplasty
    c. arthrectomy
    d. electroarthrography

13. The surgical repair of a joint is known as an
    a. arthrocentesis
    b. arthroplasty
    c. arthrectomy
    d. electroarthrography

14. The surfaces of the connecting bones are protected by a thin layer of cartilage, called the
    a. cartilage membrane
    b. articular cartilage
    c. endocartilage
    d. synovium

15. A small sac that lubricates the area around the elbow, knee, or shoulder joint where friction is most likely to occur is known as a
    a. bursa
    b. pouch
    c. articular cyst
    d. articulocele

16. An example of a hinge joint is the
    a. hip joint
    b. elbow
    c. wrist
    d. neck

17. An example of a ball-and-socket joint is the
    a. elbow
    b. knee
    c. hip joint
    d. cranial suture

18. The manual forcing of a joint back into its original position, without making an incision is known as a(n)
    a. closed reduction
    b. open reduction
    c. articulation
    d. hip pinning

19. The clicking or crackling sounds heard upon joint movement is called
    a. articulation
    b. crepitation
    c. whistles
    d. wrenching

20. The space between two connecting bones is known as the
    a. joint cavity
    b. synovial membrane
    c. bursa
    d. tendon

MATCHING

INSTRUCTIONS: Match the term on the left with the correct definition on the right. Enter your selection in the space provided.

_____ 21. flexion	a. movement that involves the turning of a bone on its own axis
_____ 22. adduction	b. movement of a bone away from the midline of the body
_____ 23. extension	c. a bending motion
_____ 24. abduction	d. a straightening motion
_____ 25. rotation	e. movement of a bone toward the midline of the body

_____ 26. supination	a. bending the foot downward at the ankle with the toes pointing downward, as in toe dancing
_____ 27. pronation	
_____ 28. dorsiflexion	b. the act of turning the palm up or forward
_____ 29. plantar flexion	c. movement of an extremity around in a circular motion
_____ 30. circumduction	d. the act of turning the palm down or backward
	e. bending the foot backward, or upward, at the ankle

_____ 31. kyphosis	a. the point of attachment of a muscle to a bone that it moves
_____ 32. malaise	b. the point of attachment of a muscle to a bone that is less movable
_____ 33. atrophy	c. humpback
_____ 34. origin	d. A vague feeling of weakness
_____ 35. insertion	e. wasting away

COMPLETION

INSTRUCTIONS: Read each statement carefully and complete the statement with the most appropriate response. Enter your answer in the space provided.

36. Pain in the joints is known as ____________________

37. An abnormal, usually permanent bending of a joint into a fixed position, usually caused by atrophy and shortening of muscle fibers is called a ____________________

38. Another name for the trunk, or main part of the body is the ____________________

39. The medical term for wasting away, literally "without development," is ____________________

40. The thin sheets of fibrous connective tissue that penetrate as well as cover the entire muscle, holding the fibers together are called ____________________

41. A joint that allows movements in many directions around a central point is known as what type of joint? ____________________

42. The thick, lubricating fluid located in synovial joints is known as ____________________

43. Inflammation of the sciatic nerve, marked by pain and tenderness along the path of the nerve through the thigh and leg is called____________________

44. The medical term viscous means ____________________

45. When an individual has an increased reaction of the skin to exposure to sunlight, he/she is said to be experiencing ____________________

46. The medical term for an incomplete dislocation is ____________________

47. Muscles that act without conscious control, being controlled by the autonomic nervous system and hormones, are known as ____________________

48. Weakness of the muscles of the pelvic girdle (the muscles that extend the hip and the knee) is often seen in individuals with muscular dystrophy, and is known as ____________________

49. Surgical removal of a bunion is known as a ____________________

50. An immovable joint is called a ____________________

CHAPTER 7 ALTERNATE COMPLETION QUESTIONS

Emphasizing Word Elements and Abbreviations

(Can be substituted for Completion Questions 36-50)

COMPLETION

INSTRUCTIONS: Read each statement carefully and complete the statement with the most appropriate response. Enter your answer in the space provided.

36. The combining form **bucc/o** means ______

37. The combining form **fasci/o** means ______

38. The combining form **fibr/o** means ______

39. The combining form **leiomy/o** means ______

40. The combining form **my/o** means ______

41. The combining form **pector/o** means ______

42. The combining form **troph/o** means ______

43. The prefix tri- means ______

44. The combining form for stiff is ______

45. The combining form that means **joint** is ______

46. The abbreviation for **left lower extremity** is ______

47. The abbreviation for **metacarpophalangeal (joint)** is ______

48. The abbreviation for **rheumatoid arthritis** is ______

49. The abbreviation for **sedimentation rate** is ______

50. The abbreviation for **systemic lupus erythematosus** is ______

CHAPTER 8 NERVOUS SYSTEM CHAPTER EXAM

MULTIPLE CHOICE

INSTRUCTIONS: The following questions or incomplete statements are followed by four answers or completions. Read each question carefully and select the most appropriate response.

1. The absence of the brain and spinal cord at birth is known as
   a. encephalopathy
   b. anencephaly
   c. hydrocephaly
   d. encephaloma
2. A temporary or permanent unilateral weakness or paralysis of the muscles in the face following trauma to the face or an unknown infection is known as
   a. Bell's palsy
   b. Parkinson's disease
   c. myasthenia gravis
   d. lupus erythematosus
3. A pinching or compression of the median nerve within the wrist area due to inflammation and swelling of the tendons, causing intermittent or continuous pain, is known as
   a. Bell's palsy
   b. Guillain-Barré syndrome
   c. carpal tunnel syndrome
   d. wrist drop
4. Another name for a stroke is
   a. cerebral concussion
   b. cerebrovascular accident
   c. cardiovascular accident
   d. encephalitis
5. A brief interruption of brain function with a loss of consciousness lasting for a few seconds, possibly due to a blow to the head, is known as a(n)
   a. cerebral contusion
   b. cerebrovascular accident
   c. encephalitis
   d. cerebral concussion
6. Inflammation of the brain or spinal cord tissue, largely caused by a virus is known as
   a. encephalitis
   b. encephalopathy
   c. encephaloma
   d. encephalocele
7. A syndrome of recurring episodes of excessive irregular electrical activity of the central nervous system (CNS) called seizures is called
   a. cerebral contusion
   b. epilepsy
   c. Bell's palsy
   d. meningitis
8. An epileptic seizure characterized by a rigid body extension and an alternating contracting and relaxing of muscles is known as a(n)
   a. petit mal seizure
   b. absence seizure
   c. grand mal seizure
   d. apoplexy
9. A small seizure in which there is a sudden, temporary loss of consciousness, lasting only a few seconds, where the individual may have a blank facial expression and may experience repeated blinking of the eyes during this brief period of time is a(n)
   a. grand mal seizure
   b. apoplexy
   c. Cheyne-Stokes respiration episode
   d. petit mal seizure
10. A recurring pulsating, vascular headache that usually develops on one side of the head and is characterized by a slow onset, and may be preceded by an *aura*, is known as a(n)
    a. migraine headache
    b. cluster headache
    c. stress headache
    d. normal headache

11. An inherited neurological disease, characterized by rapid, jerky, involuntary movements and increasing dementia due to the affects on the neurons of the basal ganglia, is known as
    a. Bell's palsy
    b. multiple sclerosis
    c. Huntington's chorea
    d. cerebral palsy

12. A congenital disorder in which there is an abnormal increase of cerebrospinal fluid in the ventricles of the brain, resulting in an increased head circumference in the infant is known as
    a. hydrocephalus
    b. hydrocele
    c. cephalalgia
    d. encephalopathy

13. A serious bacterial infection of the covering of the brain and spinal cord, that can have residual debilitating effects or even a fatal outcome if not diagnosed and treated promptly with appropriate antibiotic therapy is
    a. bacterial myitis
    b. bacterial meningitis
    c. viral hepatitis
    d. bacterial cephalitis

14. A degenerative inflammatory disease of the CNS that attacks the myelin sheath in the spinal cord and brain, leaving it scarred, is known as
    a. polyarthritis
    b. meningitis
    c. multiple sclerosis
    d. Parkinson's disease

15. A degenerative, slowly progressive, deterioration of nerves in the brain stem's motor system, characterized by a stooped posture and a shuffling gait, is known as
    a. Huntington's chorea
    b. Guillain-Barre' syndrome
    c. Parkinson's disease
    d. Bell's palsy

16. An acute viral infection seen mainly in adults characterized by inflammation of the underlying spinal or cranial nerve pathway producing painful, vesicular eruptions on the skin following along these nerve pathways is known as
    a. Reye's syndrome
    b. shingles
    c. Carpal tunnel syndrome
    d. ganglionitis

17. Paralysis of the lower extremities, as a result of severe injury to the spinal cord in the thoracic or lumbar region, is known as
    a. quadriplegia
    b. hemiplegia
    c. stroke
    d. paraplegia

18. Insertion of a hollow needle and stylet into the subarachnoid space, generally between the third and fourth lumbar vertebrae, for the purpose of withdrawing cerebrospinal fluid is a(n)
    a. lumbar puncture
    b. encephalography
    c. Romberg test
    d. spinal anesthesia

19. Visualization of the cerebral vascular system via x-ray after the injection of a radiopaque contrast medium into an arterial blood vessel (carotid, femoral, or brachial) is known as
    a. echoencephalograph
    b. cerebral angiography
    c. electroencephalography
    d. Romberg test

20. A procedure used to evaluate cerebellar function and balance, in which the person is asked to stand quietly, with eyes closed, feet together and hands at his/her side and to maintain equilibrium while responding to directions, is known as
    a. causalgia
    b. Babinski reflex
    c. Romberg testreflex
    d. Kernig's sign

MATCHING

INSTRUCTIONS: Match the term on the left with the correct definition on the right. Enter your selection in the space provided.

_____ 21. agraphia	a. without muscle coordination
_____ 22. aphasia	b. without feeling or sensation
_____ 23. analgesia	c. without sensitivity to pain
_____ 24. ataxia	d. the inability to convert one's thoughts into writing
_____ 25. anesthesia	e. inability to speak

_____ 26. aura	a. abnormally slow movement
_____ 27. axon	b. usually precedes the onset of a migraine headache or an epileptic seizure
_____ 28. dendrite	c. headache
_____ 29. bradykinesia	d. receives impulses and conducts them on to the nerve cell body
_____ 30. cephalalgia	e. transports nerve impulses away from the nerve cell body

_____ 31. central nervous system	a. transmit nerve impulses away from the central nervous system
_____ 32. autonomic nervous system	b. consists of 12 pairs of cranial nerves and 31 pairs of spinal nerves
_____ 33. peripheral nervous system	c. consists of the brain and the spinal cord
_____ 34. cerebrum	d. controls consciousness, memory, sensations, emotions, and voluntary movements
_____ 35. efferent nerves	e. regulates the involuntary vital functions of the body, such as the activities involving the heart muscle, smooth muscles, and the glands

COMPLETION

INSTRUCTIONS: Read each statement carefully and complete the statement with the most appropriate response. Enter your answer in the space provided.

36. Nerves that transmit nerve impulses toward the central nervous system are called ____________ nerves.

37. The stem-like portion of the brain that connects the cerebral hemisphere with the spinal cord is the ______________________________

38. A hole drilled into the skull using a form of drill is called a ______________________________

39. The part of the brain responsible for coordinating voluntary muscular movement is the ______________________________

40. Small scattered venous hemorrhages in the brain, described as a "bruise" of the brain tissue is known as a cerebral ______________________________

41. The fluid that flows through the brain and around the spinal cord, protecting them from physical blow or impact is known as ______________________________

42. A deep sleep in which the individual cannot be aroused and does not respond to external stimuli is known as a ______________________________

43. A surgical incision into the cranium is called a ______________________________

44. Any neurological deficiency or variation of the normal is known as a ______________________________

45. The medical term for difficult speech is ______________________________

46. Paralysis of one half of the body (left or right side) is known as ______________________________

47. Excessive sensitivity to sensory stimuli, such as pain or touch is known as ______________________________

48. The part of the brain that contains the cardiac, vasomotor, and respiratory centers, is the ______________________________

49. The three layers of protective membranes that surround the brain and spinal cord are called the ______________________________

50. The medical term for uncontrolled, sudden attacks of sleep is ______________________________

CHAPTER 8 ALTERNATE COMPLETION QUESTIONS
Emphasizing Word Elements and Abbreviations

(Can be substituted for Completion Questions 36-50)

COMPLETION

INSTRUCTIONS: Read each statement carefully and complete the statement with the most appropriate response. Enter your answer in the space provided.

36. The suffix -**algesia** means ______________________________

37. The suffix -**algia** means ______________________________

38. The prefix **brady**- means ______________________________

39. The combining form **encephal/o** means ______________________________

40. The combining form **esthesi/o** means ______________________________

41. The combining form **gli/o** means ______________________________

42. The combining form **kinesi/o** means ______________________________

43. The suffix -**lepsy** means ______________________________

44. The suffix that means **reading** is ______________________________

45. The combining form for **spinal cord** or **bone marrow** is ______________________________

46. The abbreviation for **central nervous system** is ______________________________

47. The abbreviation for a **cerebrovascular accident** is ______________________________

48. The abbreviation for an **electroencephalogram** is ______________________________

49. The abbreviation for **intracranial pressure** is ______________________________

50. The abbreviation for **positron-emission tomography** is ______________________________

CHAPTER 9 BLOOD AND LYMPHATIC SYSTEM CHAPTER EXAM

MULTIPLE CHOICE

INSTRUCTIONS: The following questions or incomplete statements are followed by four answers or completions. Read each question carefully and select the most appropriate response.

1. The abbreviation AIDS stands for
   a. autoimmune deficiency syndrome
   b. acquired immunodeficiency syndrome
   c. aplastic immunodegenerative syndrome
   d. American Immunoassay Diagnostic Standard

2. An illness caused by the Epstein-Barr virus, which is a benign, self-limiting acute infection of the B lymphocytes, occurring primarily in young adults (fifteen to twenty), and is known as the "kissing disease", is also known as
   a. strep throat
   b. mononucleosis
   c. sarcoidosis
   d. tuberculosis

3. An x-ray assessment of the lymphatic system following injection of a contrast medium into the lymph vessels in the hand or foot is known as a(n)
   a. echolymphogram
   b. renogram
   c. pyelogram
   d. lymphangiogram

4. An infectious disease, chronic in nature, primarily affecting the lungs causing large areas of cavitations and caseous ("cheeselike") necrosis, that is spread through droplet infection is known as
   a. AIDS
   b. tuberculosis
   c. syphilis
   d. mononucleosis

5. A malignant neoplasm of the blood vessels, associated with AIDS, characterized by lesions appearing initially as tiny red to purple macules and evolving into sizable modules or plaques is known as
   a. Kaposi's sarcoma
   b. malignant melanoma
   c. astrocytoma
   d. purpura

6. A form of anemia that is due to a lack of Vitamin B_{12} absorption that is necessary for the proper maturation of the red blood cells is
   a. aplastic anemia
   b. sickle cell anemia
   c. pernicious anemia
   d. hemolytic anemia

7. A chronic hereditary form of hemolytic anemia in which the RBCs become shaped like a crescent in the presence of low oxygen concentration is
   a. aplastic anemia
   b. sickle cell anemia
   c. pernicious anemia
   d. hemolytic anemia

8. A term used to define different hereditary deficiencies of coagulation factors, such as Factor VIII, that result in prolonged bleeding times is known as
   a. pancytopenia
   b. purpura
   c. sarcoidosis
   d. hemophilia

9. A malignancy of the blood forming cells in the bone marrow, characterized by excessive uncontrolled increase of immature WBCs in the blood eventually leading to infection, anemia, and thrombocytopenia, is known as
   a. leukemia
   b. purpura
   c. sarcoidosis
   d. hemophilia

10. A collection of small hemorrhages beneath the skin, appearing as red-purple skin discolorations, is caused from a decreased number of circulating platelets, and is known as
    a. leukocytopenia
    b. purpura
    c. eczema
    d. hemangiitis

11. A blood test used for screening for an antibody to the AIDS virus is
    a. ELISA
    b. AFB
    c. Direct Coombs
    d. ESR

12. An abnormal proliferation of RBCs, granulocytes, and thrombocytes leading to an increase in blood volume and viscosity (thickness) is known as
    a. purpura
    b. polycythemia vera
    c. hemochromatosis
    d. thalassemia

13. Measurement of the time that is required for bleeding to stop (normally one to nine minutes) is known as
    a. clotting time
    b. sedimentation rate
    c. bleeding time
    d. bleed through

14. Administration of blood or a blood component to an individual in order to replace blood lost through surgery, trauma, or disease is known as a(n)
    a. bleed through
    b. blood transfusion
    c. hemodialysis
    d. blood purge

15. The test that measures the settling distance of red blood cells in normal saline over a one hour period of time is known as
    a. hemolysis rate
    b. complete blood cell count
    c. red blood cell count
    d. erythrocyte sedimentation rate

16. When people receive blood or a blood component that has been previously collected from themselves through a reinfusion it is called a(n)
    a. autologous transfusion
    b. blood purge
    c. biological transfusion
    d. hemodialysis exchange

17. The test that is an assessment of red blood cell percentage in the total blood volume is known as
    a. erythrocyte sedimentation rate
    b. hematocrit
    c. hemoglobin
    d. blood smear

18. An examination of the RBC on a stained blood smear that enables the examiner to identify the form and shape of the RBCs is known as
    a. reticuloblastocyte count
    b. red blood cell morphology
    c. erythroblastocyte count
    d. cell differential

19. The measurement of the percentage of each specific type of circulating WBCs present in the one cubic millimeter of peripheral blood is known as a
    a. white blood cell differential
    b. white blood cell metamorphosis
    c. white blood cell reticulocyte count
    d. white blood cell roleaux

20. A diagnostic analysis for pernicious anemia is the
    a. rouleux
    b. Schilling test
    c. Romberg test
    d. reticulocyte count

MATCHING

INSTRUCTIONS: Match the term on the left with the correct definition on the right. Enter your selection in the space provided.

_____ 21. agglutination
_____ 22. anaphylaxis
_____ 23. dyscrasia
_____ 24. erythrocyte
_____ 25. erythropoietin

a. a mature red blood cell
b. stimulates and regulates the production of erythrocytes
c. clumping together of cells as a result of interaction with specific antibodies called agglutinins
d. any abnormal condition of the blood or bone marrow
e. an exaggerated, life threatening hypersensitivity reaction to a previously encountered antigen.

_____ 26. leukocytopenia
_____ 27. plasma
_____ 28. platelet
_____ 29. serum
_____ 30. thrombus

a. the clear, thin, and sticky fluid portion of the blood that remains after coagulation
b. a clotting cell
c. a clot
d. an abnormal decrease in number of white blood cells
e. the watery, straw-colored, fluid portion of the lymph and the blood

_____ 31. edema
_____ 32. immunity
_____ 33. pathogens
_____ 34. aplastic
_____ 35. hemolytic

a. a form of anemia in which there is a failure of all blood cells to develop
b. the state of being resistant to or protected from a disease
c. a form of anemia characterized by extreme reduction in circulating red blood cells due to their destruction
d. the accumulation of fluid within the tissue spaces
e. disease-producing microorganisms

COMPLETION

INSTRUCTIONS: Read each statement carefully and complete the statement with the most appropriate response. Enter your answer in the space provided.

36. A substance that can produce a hypersensitive reaction in the body but is not necessarily harmful is called a(n) ______________________________

37. The process of transforming a liquid into a solid, especially of the blood, is called ______________________________

38. The abnormal accumulation of fluid in interstitial spaces of tissues is known as ______________________

39. A marked reduction in the number of red blood cells, white blood cells, and platelets, is known as ______________________

40. A systemic infection in which pathogens are present in the circulating bloodstream is known as ______________________

41. An abnormal enlargement of the spleen is called ______________________

42. A platelet is also called a ______________________

43. Another name for a clot is a ______________________

44. A dislodged, circulating clot is known as an ______________________

45. A substance, usually a protein, that causes the formation of an antibody and reacts specifically with that antibody is known as a(n) ______________________

46. Immunity that is a result of the body's developing the ability to defend itself against a specific agent, as a result of having had the disease or from having received an immunization against a disease, is known as ______________________

47. Immunity with which we are born; also called genetic immunity is known as ______________________

48. Disease-producing microorganisms are called ______________________

49. When an individual is in a state of having a lack of resistance to pathogens and other harmful agents, the individual is said to be ______________________

50. A reaction to treatment that occurs at the site of administration is known as a ______________________ reaction.

CHAPTER 9 ALTERNATE COMPLETION QUESTIONS

Emphasizing Word Elements and Abbreviations

(Can be substituted for Completion Questions 36-50)

COMPLETION

INSTRUCTIONS: Read each statement carefully and complete the statement with the most appropriate response. Enter your answer in the space provided.

36. The combining form **agglutin/o** means ______________________________

37. The combining form **chrom/o** means ______________________________

38. The combining form **cyt/o** means ______________________________

39. The suffix -**emia** means ______________________________

40. The combining form **eosin/o** means ______________________________

41. The suffix -**stasis** means ______________________________

42. One of the combining forms for **blood** is ______________________________

43. The combining form **morph/o** means ______________________________

44. The suffix that means **deficiency** is ______________________________

45. The suffix that means **to eat** is ______________________________

46. The abbreviation for **complete blood(cell) count** is ______________________________

47. An abbreviation for **hemoglobin** is ______________________________

48. The abbreviation for **hematocrit** is ______________________________

49. The abbreviation for **communicable disease center** is ______________________________

50. The abbreviation for **human immunodeficiency virus** is ______________________________

CHAPTER 10 CARDIOVASCULAR SYSTEM CHAPTER EXAM

MULTIPLE CHOICE

INSTRUCTIONS: The following questions or incomplete statements are followed by four answers or completions. Read each question carefully and select the most appropriate response.

1. The medical name for a heart attack is
   a. angina
   b. myocardial infarction
   c. myocarditis
   d. myocardiopathy

2. A condition in which the heart is unable to pump effectively is characterized by weakness, breathlessness, abdominal discomfort, congestion, and edema in the lower portions of the body. This condition is known as
   a. congestive heart failure
   b. myocarditis
   c. click-murmur syndrome
   d. myocardial infarction

3. Inflammation of the membrane lining the valves and chambers of the heart is known as
   a. myocarditis
   b. cardiomyopathy
   c. endocarditis
   d. pancarditis

4. An inflammatory disease, usually occuring in children ages 5 to 15, that may develop as a delayed reaction to an insufficiently treated Group A beta-hemolytic streptococcal infection of the upper respiratory tract is known as
   a. mitral valve prolapse
   b. rheumatic fever
   c. angina pectoris
   d. Raynaud's phenomenon

5. Inflammation of the saclike membrane that covers the heart muscle is known as
   a. endocarditis
   b. rheumatic fever
   c. cardiomyopathy
   d. pericarditis

6. Mitral valve prolapse is also known as
   a. click-murmur syndrome
   b. Raynaud's phenomenon
   c. congestive heart failure
   d. Sydenham's chorea

7. A localized dilatation of an artery formed at a weak point in the vessel wall, that balloons out with each pulsation of the artery is called a(n)
   a. herniation
   b. varicosity
   c. aneurysm
   d. hydrocele

8. An arterial condition in which there is thickening, hardening, and loss of elasticity of the walls of arteries, resulting in decreased blood supply, especially to the lower extremities and cerebrum is known as
   a. arteriosclerosis
   b. thrombophlebitis
   c. varicose veins
   d. petechia

9. Inflammation of a vein associated with the formation of a thrombus (clot) is called
   a. arteriosclerosis
   b. thrombophlebitis
   c. varicose veins
   d. petechia

10. The form of hypertension that accounts for approximately 90% of all hypertension and has no single known cause is known as
    a. malignant hypertension
    b. dependent hypertension
    c. secondary hypertension
    d. essential hypertension

11. Hypertension that is caused by complications of another condition such as pregnancy or kidney disease is known as
    a. malignant hypertension
    b. dependent hypertension
    c. secondary hypertension
    d. essential hypertension

12. A term given to hypertension that is severe and rapidly progressive, characterized by a diastolic pressure higher than 120 mm Hg., severe headaches, confusion, and blurred vision, is
    a. malignant hypertension
    b. dependent hypertension
    c. secondary hypertension
    d. essential hypertension

13. Intermittent attacks of vasoconstriction of the arterioles, causing pallor of the fingers or toes, followed by cyanosis, then redness, before returning to normal color is known as
    a. mitral valve prolapse
    b. diaphoresis
    c. angina pectoris
    d. Raynaud's phenomenon

14. A condition in which the contractions of the atria become extremely rapid, at the rate of between 250 to 400 beats per minute is known as
    a. atrial fibrillation
    b. atrial flutter
    c. ventricular fibrillation
    d. ventricullar flutter

15. A condition characterized by extremely rapid, incomplete contractions of the atria resulting in disorganized and uncoordinated twitching of the atria, with the rate of contractions being as high as 350 to 600 beats per minute is known as
    a. atrial fibrillation
    b. atrial flutter
    c. ventricular fibrillation
    d. ventricullar flutter

16. A graphic record (visual representation) of the electrical action of the heart as reflected from various angles to the surface of the skin is known as a(n)
    a. echocardiogram
    b. electrocardiogram
    c. endocardiograph
    d. cardiac MRI

17. A small, portable monitoring devise that makes prolonged electrocardiograph recordings on a portable tape recorder is known as a
    a. Holter monitor
    b. halter monitor
    c. sonogram
    d. portable echocardiograph

18. An abnormal sound or murmur heard when listening to a carotid artery, organ, or gland with a stethoscope; i.e., during auscultation is known as a(n)
    a. bruit
    b. murmur
    c. claudication
    d. rale

19. Cramp-like pains in the calves of the legs caused by poor circulation to the muscles of the legs, commonly associated with atherosclerosis, are known as
    a. varicosities
    b. bruits
    c. claudication
    d. tetany

20. A form of arteriosclerosis (hardening of the arteries) characterized by fatty deposits building up within the inner layers of the walls of larger arteries is known as
    a. atherosclerosis
    b. coronary arteritis
    c. Sydenham's chorea
    d. vegetations

MATCHING

INSTRUCTIONS: Match the term on the left with the correct definition on the right. Enter your selection in the space provided.

_____ 21. fatigue
_____ 22. dyspnea
_____ 23. fever
_____ 24. weakness
_____ 25. pallor

a. lacking physical strength or vigor.
b. lack of color; paleness
c. a feeling of tiredness or weariness resulting from continued activity or as a side effect from some psychotropic disease
d. elevation of temperature above the normal
e. air hunger resulting in labored or difficult breathing, sometimes accompanied by pain

_____ 26. tachycardia
_____ 27. bradycardi
_____ 28. palpitation
_____ 29. cyanosis
_____ 30. sweat

a. rapid, violent, or throbbing pulsation, as an abnormally rapid throbbing or fluttering of the heart, felt by the patient
b. perspiration
c. abnormal rapidity of heart action, usually defined as a heart rate over 100 beats per minute
d. slightly bluish, grayish, slatelike, or dark discoloration of the skin
e. a slow heart rate that is characterized by a pulse rate that is under 60 beats per minute

_____ 31. nausea
_____ 32. anorexia
_____ 33. vomiting
_____ 34. pitting edema
_____ 35. dependent edema

a. swelling, usually of the skin of the extremities, that when pressed firmly with a finger will maintain the dent produced by the finger
b. unpleasant sensation usually preceding vomiting
c. loss of appetite
d. ejection through the mouth of the gastric contents
e. a fluid accumulation in the tissues influenced by gravity; usually greater in the lower extremities than in tissue levels above the level of the heart

COMPLETION

INSTRUCTIONS: Read each statement carefully and complete the statement with the most appropriate response. Enter your answer in the space provided.

36. A localized dilation of a weakened area of the wall of an artery is known as a(n)

____

37. Any one of the small flaps on the valves of the heart is known as a _______________________

38. The period of relaxation of the heart, alternating with the contraction phase, is known as the

____

39. A dysrhythmia is an ______________________________

40. Inflammation of the inner lining of the heart is known as ______________________________

41. The medical term for low blood pressure, or less than normal blood pressure readings is ______________________________

42. The area between the lungs, in the chest cavity, that contains the heart, aorta, trachea, esophagus, and bronchi, is known as the ______________________________

43. The only arteries in the body that transport de-oxygenated blood are the ______________________________

44. The SA node of the heart is also known as the ______________________________ of the heart.

45. The circulation of the blood from the left ventricle of the heart, throughout the body, and back to the right atrium of the heart is known as ______________________________ circulation.

46. The circulation of deoxygenated blood from the right ventricle of the heart to the lungs for oxygenation and back to the left atrium of the heart is known as ______________________________ circulation.

47. The contraction phase of the heart beat, forcing blood into the aorta and the pulmonary arteries is known as ______________________________

48. Narrowing of the lumen of a blood vessel is called ______________________________

49. An abnormal growth of tissue around a valve is called a(n) ______________________________

50. The medical term for high blood pressure is ______________________________

CHAPTER 10 ALTERNATE COMPLETION QUESTIONS
Emphasizing Word Elements and Abbreviations

(Can be substituted for Completion Questions 36-50)

COMPLETION

INSTRUCTIONS: Read each statement carefully and complete the statement with the most appropriate response. Enter your answer in the space provided.

36. The combining form **angi/o** means ____________________

37. The combining form **ather/o** means ____________________

38. The combining form **cardi/o** means ____________________

39. The combining form **coron/o** means ____________________

40. The combining form **ech/o** means ____________________

41. The combining form **electr/o** means ____________________

42. The prefix **endo-** means ____________________

43. The combining form **graph/o** means ____________________

44. The combining form that means **enlarged** is ____________________

45. The combining form for **muscle** is ____________________

46. The abbreviation for **bundle branch block** is____________________

47. The abbreviation for **arteriosclerotic heart disease** is ____________________

48. The abbreviation for **hypertensive cardiovascular disease** is ____________________

49. The abbreviation for **congestive heart failure** is ____________________

50. The abbreviation for **myocardial infarction** or **heart attack** is ____________________

CHAPTER 11 RESPIRATORY SYSTEM CHAPTER EXAM

MULTIPLE CHOICE

INSTRUCTIONS: The following questions or incomplete statements are followed by four answers or completions. Read each question carefully and select the most appropriate response.

1. The functional units of the lungs are the
   a. alveoli
   b. bronchi
   c. bronchioles
   d. pleura
2. A productive cough is one that
   a. is dry and irritating, forcing the individual to cough
   b. is tickling to the throat
   c. is effective in bringing up sputum
   d. has hacking sound
3. The medical term for a nosebleed is
   a. epistaxis
   b. rhinitis
   c. rhinorrhea
   d. hemoptysis
4. The act of spitting out saliva or coughing up materials from the air passageways leading to the lungs is called
   a. hemoptysis
   b. rhinorrhea
   c. expectoration
   d. stridor
5. Expectoration of blood arising from the oral cavity, larynx, trachea, bronchi, or lungs is known as
   a. hemoptysis
   b. rhinorrhea
   c. expectoration
   d. stridor
6. A thin watery discharge from the nose is known as
   a. hemoptysis
   b. rhinorrhea
   c. rhinitis
   d. sinusitis
7. An abnormal sound heard on auscultation of the chest, that is a cracking sound similar to that of moisture crackling in a tube as air passes through it is known as
   a. bruits
   b. rhonchi
   c. rales
   d. murmurs
8. A harsh sound during respiration, particularly inhalation, that is high-pitched and resembles the blowing of wind, due to obstruction of air passages is known as
   a. bruit
   b. rales
   c. rhonchi
   d. stridor
9. A whistling sound resulting from narrowing of the lumen of a respiratory passageway, heard without the aid of a stethoscope, usually during exhalation is known as
   a. stridor
   b. wheezing
   c. bruits
   d. dysphonia
10. Difficulty in speaking, or hoarseness is known as
    a. stridor
    b. dysphagia
    c. dysphonia
    d. dyspnea

11. Temporary cessation of breathing is termed
    a. dyspnea
    b. bradypnea
    c. tachypnea
    d. apnea
12. Breathing in any but erect, sitting or standing position is known as
    a. dyspnea
    b. orthopnea
    c. apnea
    d. bradypnea
13. Abnormal rapidity of breathing is known as
    a. dyspnea
    b. bradypnea
    c. tachypnea
    d. apnea
14. Abnormally slow breathing is known as
    a. dyspnea
    b. bradypnea
    c. tachypnea
    d. apnea
15. A very deep gasping type of respiration associated with severe diabetic acidosis is known as
    a. stridoric respirations
    b. shallow respirations
    c. Kussmaul's respirations
    d. dyspnea
16. Inflammation of the respiratory mucous membranes known as the common cold is
    a. coryza
    b. sinusitis
    c. pharyngitis
    d. allergic rhinitis
17. A childhood disease characterized by a barking cough, suffocative and difficult breathing, stridor, and laryngeal spasm is
    a. croup
    b. pneumonia
    c. pleurisy
    d. tuberculosis
18. Pus in a body cavity, especially in the pleural cavity (pyothorax) that is usually the result of a primary infection in the lungs is known as
    a. emphysema
    b. empyema
    c. pleurisy
    d. pneumonia
19. A collection of air or gas in the pleural cavity, as the result of a perforation through the chest wall or the pleura covering the lung (visceral pleura) is known as
    a. pulmonary embolism
    b. pulmonary edema
    c. pulmonary infarct
    d. pneumothorax
20. The use of a needle to collect pleural fluid for laboratory analysis, or to remove excess pleural fluid or air from the pleural space is known as a(n)
    a. bronchoscopy
    b. thoracentesis
    c. abdominocentesis
    d. pleural effusion

MATCHING

INSTRUCTIONS: Match the term on the left with the correct definition on the right. Enter your selection in the space provided.

_____ 21. inspection
_____ 22. palpation
_____ 23. auscultation
_____ 24. percussion
_____ 25. bronchoscopy

a. examination of the interior of the bronchi using a lighted, flexible, endoscope
b. use of the fingertips to tap the body lightly but sharply to determine position, size, and consistency of an underlying structure and the presence of fluid or pus in a cavity
c. process of examining by application of the hands or fingers to the external surface of the body
d. process of listening, with a stethoscope, for sounds within the body
e. visual examination of the external surface of the body as well as of its movements and posture

_____ 26. anthracosis
_____ 27. asbestosis
_____ 28. byssinosis
_____ 29. silicosis
_____ 30. pleurisy

a. Brown Lung Disease
b. a lung disease resulting from inhalation of silica (quartz) dust
c. inflammation of both the visceral and parietal pleura
d. a lung disease resulting from inhalation of asbestos particles
e. Black Lung Disease

_____ 31. lung cancer
_____ 32. cor pulmonale
_____ 33. asthma
_____ 34. emphysema
_____ 35. pulmonary edema

a. a chronic pulmonary disease in which the lungs lose their elasticity
b. swelling of the lungs caused by an abnormal accumulation of fluid in the lungs, either in alveoli or the interstitial spaces
c. pulmonary heart disease
d. paryoxysmal dyspnea accompanied by wheezing
e. bronchiogenic carcinoma

COMPLETION

INSTRUCTIONS: Read each statement carefully and complete the statement with the most appropriate response. Enter your answer in the space provided.

36. The upper portion of the lung, rising just above the collarbone is known as the _____________________

37. The lower portion of the lung, that rests on the diaphragm, is known as the _____________________

38. Another name for the larynx is the _____________________

39. Another name for the trachea is the _____________________

40. The part of the pharynx located above the soft palate in the postnasal space is known as the _____________________

41. The double folded membrane that lines the thoracic cavity is the _____________________

42. Another name for the thorax is the ______________________________

43. Another name for the pharynx is the ______________________________

44. The external nostrils are called the ______________________________

45. The thin, leaf-shaped structure that covers the entrance of the larynx when the individual swallows is the ______________________________

46. The musculomembranous wall that separates the abdominal and thoracic cavities, and aids in the process of respiration is the ______________________________

47. The two main branches leading from the trachea to the lungs are the ______________________________

48. The functional units of the lungs are the ______________________________

49. The hollow areas or cavities within the skull that communicate with the nasal cavity are known as the ______________________________

50. The portion of the pleura that is closest to the internal organs is the ______________________________ pleura.

CHAPTER 11 ALTERNATE COMPLETION QUESTIONS

Emphasizing Word Elements and Abbreviations

(Can be substituted for Completion Questions 36-50)

COMPLETION

INSTRUCTIONS: Read each statement carefully and complete the statement with the most appropriate response. Enter your answer in the space provided.

36. The combining form **alveol/o** means ______________________________

37. The combining form **bronch/o** means ______________________________

38. The combining form **laryng/o** means ______________________________

39. The combining form **pector/o** means ______________________________

40. The combining form **phren/o** means ______________________________

41. The combining form **pulmon/o** means ______________________________

42. The combining form **pne/o** means ______________________________

43. The combining form **pneumon/o** means ______________________________

44. One combining form for **nose** is ______________________________

45. A combining form, other than pector/o, for **chest** is ______________________________

46. The abbreviation **SOB** stands for ______________________________

47. The abbreviation **SIDS** stands for______________________________

48. The abbreviation **LLL** stands for ______________________________

49. The abbreviation **IPPB** stands for ______________________________

50. The abbreviation **COPD** stands for ______________________________

CHAPTER 12 DIGESTIVE SYSTEM CHAPTER EXAM

MULTIPLE CHOICE

INSTRUCTIONS: The following questions or incomplete statements are followed by four answers or completions. Read each question carefully and select the most appropriate response.

1. An abnormal passageway in the skin surface near the anus usually connecting with the rectum is known as a(n)
   a. anal ulcer
   b. anal fistula
   c. rectal ulcer
   d. anocele
2. A condition in which the individual has small inflammatory non-infectious ulcerated lesions occurring on the lips, tongue, and inside the cheeks of the mouth is
   a. aphthous stomatitis
   b. pyorrhea
   c. chronic polyposis
   d. Crohn's disease
3. A chronic digestive tract inflammation that causes fever, cramping, diarrhea, weight loss, anorexia, and extreme swelling of the bowel and can lead to an obstruction is known as
   a. chronic polyposis
   b. Crohn's disease
   c. a peptic ulcer
   d. an intestinal virus
4. Another name for tooth decay caused by acid-forming microorganisms is
   a. pyorrhea
   b. gingivitis
   c. dental caries
   d. aphthous stomatitis
5. Pigmented or hardened cholesterol stones formed as a result of bile crystallization are known as
   a. gallstones
   b. renal calculi
   c. kidney stones
   d. lipid stones
6. Permanently distended veins in the distal rectum or anus are known as
   a. rectal polyps
   b. hemorrhoids
   c. rectoceles
   d. rectal phlebitis
7. An acute or chronic inflammation of the liver due to a viral or bacterial infection, drugs, alcohol, toxins, or parasites, in which the individual experiences symptoms such as abdominal and gastric discomfort, enlarged tender liver, jaundice, anorexia, and joint pain, is
   a. stomatitis
   b. pancreatitis
   c. hepatitis
   d. biliary obstruction
8. An irregular protrusion of tissue, organ, or a portion of an organ through an abnormal break in the surrounding cavity's muscular wall is a(n)
   a. hernia
   b. polyp
   c. calculus
   d. varicosity
9. Increased motility of the small or large intestinal wall resulting in abdominal pain, flatulence, nausea, anorexia and the trapping of gas throughout the intestines is known as
   a. Crohn's disease
   b. irritable bowel syndrome
   c. intestinal polyps
   d. anal fistulas
10. A fungal infection in the mouth and throat producing sore, creamy white, slightly raised curdlike patches on the tongue and other oral mucosal surfaces, that is caused by Candida albicans is known as
   a. thrush
   b. oral leukoplakia
   c. pyorrhea
   d. gingivitis

11. The insertion of a needle or trochar into the peritoneal cavity to remove excess fluid is known as a(n)
    a. thoracentesis
    b. thoracotomy
    c. abdominotomy
    d. abdominocentesis

12. The surgical creation of a new opening on the abdominal wall through which the feces will be expelled by bringing the incised colon out to the abdominal surface is known as a
    a. abdominostomy
    b. colotomy
    c. colostomy
    d. fecostomy

13. Visualization of the gallbladder through x-ray following the oral ingestion of pills containing a radiopaque iodinated dye is known as a(n)
    a. oral cholecystography
    b. fluoroscopy
    c. cholecystectomy
    d. oral colography

14. The surgical removal of the gallbladder is known as a
    a. colostomy
    b. cystectomy
    c. cholectomy
    d. cholecystectomy

15. The irrigation, or washing out of the stomach, with sterile water or a saline solution, is known as a
    a. gastric lavage
    b. coloclysis
    c. saline bath
    d. stomatoclysis

16. A term to describe the surgical repair of a hernia by closing the defect using sutures, mesh, or wire is known as a
    a. herniorrhotomy
    b. herniorrectomy
    c. herniorrhaphy
    d. herniopexy

17. X-rays of the small intestine, taken at timed intervals to observe the progression of a contrast medium, barium sulfate, through the small intestine is known as
    a. upper G.I. series
    b. intestinal lavage
    c. gastroscopy
    d. small bowel follow through

18. A back flow of contents of the stomach into the esophagus that is often the result of incompetence of the lower esophageal sphincter is known as
    a. gastroesophageal reflux
    b. nausea
    c. belching
    d. borborygmus

19. Another name for jaundice is
    a. exanthemia
    b. icterus
    c. biliariosis
    d. pallor

20. An audible abdominal sound produced by hyperactive intestinal peristalsis that can be heard, when listening with a stethoscope, as a rumbling, gurgling, or tinkling sound is known as
    a. achalasia
    b. diverticulitis
    c. borborygmus
    d. Crohn's disease

MATCHING

INSTRUCTIONS: Match the term on the left with the correct definition on the right. Enter your selection in the space provided.

_____ 21. achlorhydria	a. excessive leanness caused by disease or lack of nutrition
_____ 22. aphagia	b. a vague feeling of epigastric discomfort felt after eating
_____ 23. ascites	c. an abnormal condition characterized by the absence of hydrochloric acid in the gastric juice
_____ 24. dyspepsia	d. a condition characterized by the loss of the ability to swallow
_____ 25. emaciation	e. an abnormal accumulation of fluid within the peritoneal cavity

_____ 26. emesis	a. air or gas in the intestine that is passed through the rectum
_____ 27. eructation	b. a common chronic condition of itching of the skin around the anus
_____ 28. flatulence	c. an unpleasant sensation often leading to the urge to vomit
_____ 29. nausea	d. the material expelled from the stomach during vomiting
_____ 30. pruritus ani	e. the act of bringing up air from the stomach, through the mouth, with a characteristic sound

_____ 31. steatorrhea	a. the passage of digested food molecules into intestinal cells
_____ 32. vomitus	b. swallowing
_____ 33. absorption	c. greater than normal amounts of fat in the feces
_____ 34. mastication	d. emesis
_____ 35. deglutition	e. chewing

COMPLETION

INSTRUCTIONS: Read each statement carefully and complete the statement with the most appropriate response. Enter your answer in the space provided.

36. An enzyme that breaks down starch into smaller carbohydrate molecules is ________________________

37. A bitter, yellow-green secretion of the liver is ____

38. A medical doctor who specializes in the study of the diseases and disorders affecting the gastrointestinal tract, including the stomach, intestines, gallbladder, and bile duct is known as a ____________________

39. The liquid-like material, of partially digested food and digestive secretions, found in the stomach just before it is released into the duodenum is called ______________________________________

40. The part of the tooth that is visible above the gum line is the ______________________

41. The first set of primary teeth, or "baby teeth", are known as the ______________________

42. The act of expelling feces from the rectum through the anus is known as ______________________

43. An allied health professional trained to plan nutrition programs for sick as well as healthy people is known as a ______________________

44. The process of altering the chemical and physical composition of food so that it can be utilized by the body cells is called ______________________

45. The hard white substance that covers the dentin of the crown of a tooth is ______________________

46. A gland that secretes its enzymes directly into the blood capillaries instead of being transported via ducts is known as a(n) ______________________

47. A gland that secretes its enzymes into a network of tiny ducts that transport it to the surface of an organ or tissue or into a vessel is known as a(n) ______________________

48. A procedure in which liquid or semi-liquid food is introduced into the stomach through a tube is known as a ______________________

49. Another name for the gums is ______________________

50. A hormone, produced by the alpha cells of the pancreas, that stimulates the liver to convert glycogen into glucose when the blood sugar level is dangerously low is ______________________

CHAPTER 12 ALTERNATE COMPLETION QUESTIONS

Emphasizing Word Elements and Abbreviations

(Can be substituted for Completion Questions 36-50)

COMPLETION

INSTRUCTIONS: Read each statement carefully and complete the statement with the most appropriate response. Enter your answer in the space provided.

36. The combining form **amyl/o** means ______________________________

37. The suffix **-ase** means ______________________________

38. The combining form **bil/i** means ______________________________

39. The combining form **cheil/o** means ______________________________

40. The suffix **-ectasia** means ______________________________

41. The suffix **-emesis** means ______________________________

42. The combining form **enter/o** means ______________________________

43. The combining form **stomat/o** means ______________________________

44. The combining form for **gums** is ______________________________

45. The combining form for **tongue** is ______________________________

46. The combining form for **liver** is______________________________

47. The combining form for **stomach** is ______________________________

48. The suffix that means **perforation** is ______________________________

49. The combining form for **sigmoid colon** is ______________________________

50. The combining form for **saliva** is ______________________________

CHAPTER 13 ENDOCRINE SYSTEM CHAPTER EXAM

MULTIPLE CHOICE

INSTRUCTIONS: The following questions or incomplete statements are followed by four answers or completions. Read each question carefully and select the most appropriate response.

1. A chronic metabolic condition characterized by gradual noticeable enlargement and elongation of the bones of the face, jaw, and extremities, due to over secretion of the pituitary gland after puberty is known as
   a. acromegaly
   b. adenopathy
   c. gigantism
   d. dwarfism

2. A condition occurring in pregnancy that is characterized by signs and symptoms such as impaired ability to metabolize carbohydrates due to insulin deficiency, and elevated blood sugar level is known as
   a. diabetes insipidus
   b. diabetes mellitus
   c. gestational diabetes
   d. cretinism

3. A condition due to a deficiency in the secretion of antidiuretic hormone (ADH) by the posterior pituitary gland, characterized by large amounts of urine and sodium being excreted from the body is known as
   a. diabetes mellitus
   b. diabetes insipidus
   c. gestational diabetes
   d. cretinism

4. Generalized growth retardation of the body due to the deficiency of the human growth hormone is known as
   a. dwarfism
   b. gigantism
   c. cretinism
   d. acromegaly

5. A proportional overgrowth of the body's tissue due to the hypersecretion of the human growth hormone before puberty, causing the child to experience accelerated abnormal growth chiefly in the long bones is known as
   a. dwarfism
   b. gigantism
   c. cretinism
   d. acromegaly

6. Hyperplasia of the thyroid gland, that results from a deficient amount of iodine in the diet, is known as
   a. simple, non-toxic goiter
   b. exophthalmia
   c. thyroid storm
   d. acromegaly

7. The most severe form of hypothyroidism characterized by a puffy appearance and a thick tongue is
   a. myxedema
   b. acromegaly
   c. Cushing's syndrome
   d. thyrotoxicosis

8. Grave's disease is also known as
   a. hypothyroidism
   b. hyperthyroidism
   c. acromegaly
   d. diabetes insipidus

9. Thyrotoxicosis is also known as
   a. myxedema
   b. thyroid storm
   c. acromegaly
   d. Cushing's syndrome

10. The adrenal gland condition that includes symptoms such as central obesity, round "moon" face, edema, hypertension, "buffalo hump", muscular weakness and wasting, edema, skin infection, poor wound healing, low potassium level, and emotional changes, is known as
    a. Cushing's syndrome
    b. thyrotoxicosis
    c. Addison's disease
    d. acromegaly

11. A life threatening adrenal cortex disease that includes symptoms such as low blood glucose, low blood sodium, weight loss, dehydration, generalized weakness, gastrointestinal disturbances, increased pigmentation of the skin and mucous membranes, cold intolerance, anxiety, and depression, is known as
    a. Cushing's syndrome
    b. Addison's disease
    c. virilism
    d. thyrotoxicosis

12. A disorder of the pancreas in which the beta cells of the Islets of Langerhans of the pancreas fail to produce an adequate amount of insulin, resulting in the body's inability to appropriately metabolize carbohydrates, fats, and proteins is known as
    a. Addison's disease
    b. diabetes insipidus
    c. diabetes mellitus
    d. Cushing's syndrome

13. The classic symptoms of the disease identified in question # 12 are
    1. polydipsia
    2. glycosuria
    3. dehydration
    4. polyuria
    5. low sodium blood level

    a. 1,3,5
    b. 1,2,4
    c. 2,3,4,5
    d. 1,2,3,4,5

14. Development of male secondary sex characteristics in the female due to the excessive secretion of adrenocortical androgens from the adrenal cortex is known as
    a. virilism
    b. hyperparathyroidism
    c. cretinism
    d. Cushing's syndrome

15. Another name for the anterior pituitary gland is the
    a. neurohypophysis
    b. pituitary cortex
    c. adenohypophysis
    d. adrenocortex

16. A congenital condition caused by a lack of thyroid secretion, that is characterized by dwarfism, slowed mental development, puffy facial features, dry skin, and large tongue is known as
    a. cretinism
    b. adenopathy
    c. gigantism
    d. dwarfism

17. A ductless gland that produces a chemical substance called a hormone, that is secreted directly into the bloodstream instead of exiting the body through ducts is known as a(n)
    a. exocrine gland
    b. adenoma
    c. endocrine gland
    d. hormogenic

18. An abnormal condition characterized by a marked outward protrusion of the eyeballs is known as
    a. euthyroid
    b. exophthalmia
    c. gigantism
    d. virilism

19. A test that evaluates the person's ability to tolerate a concentrated oral glucose load by measuring the glucose levels prior to glucose administration, thirty minutes, one hour, two hours, and three hours later is known as a(n)
    a. glucose tolerance test
    b. fasting blood sugar
    c. thyroid scan
    d. glucolysis analysis

20. A disease that occurs as a consequence of long-term diabetes mellitus in which the capillaries of the retina of the eye experience microaneurysms, hemorrhages, and scarring, is known as
    a. diabetic exophthalmia
    b. arteriosclerosis
    c. diabetic retinopathy
    d. optic diabetolysis

MATCHING

INSTRUCTIONS: Match the term on the left with the correct definition on the right. Enter your selection in the space provided.

_____ 21. endocrinologist	a. an elevated blood potassium level
_____ 22. euthyroid	b. the presence of sugar in the urine
_____ 23. glycosuria	c. elevated blood calcium level
_____ 24. hypercalcemia	d. a physician who specializes in the medical practice of treating the diseases and disorders of the endocrine system
_____ 25. hyperkalemia	e. pertaining to a normally functioning thyroid gland

_____ 26. glycogenesis	a. the conversion of excess glucose into glycogen for storage in the liver for later use as needed
_____ 27. hyperglycemia	b. also called Grave's disease
_____ 28. hypernatremia	c. less than normal blood calcium level
_____ 29. hyperthyroidism	d. elevated blood sugar level
_____ 30. hypocalcemia	e. an elevated blood sodium level

_____ 31. hypoglycemia	a. the excretion of excessively large amounts of urine
_____ 32. hypokalemia	b. less than normal blood sugar level
_____ 33. hyponatremia	c. less than normal blood potassium level
_____ 34. insulin shock	d. less than normal blood sodium level
_____ 35. polyuria	e. a state of shock due to extremely low blood sugar level

COMPLETION

INSTRUCTIONS: Read each statement carefully and complete the statement with the most appropriate response. Enter your answer in the space provided.

36. The internal part of a structure organ is known as the ______________________________

37. The sum of all physical and chemical processes that take place within the body is known as ______________________________

38. The medical term for excessive thirst is ______________________________

39. A hormone secreted by the posterior pituitary gland that stimulates the contractions of the uterus during chilbirth and stimulates the release of milk from the breasts of lactating women is ______________________________

40. The somatotropic hormone is also called the ______________________________

41. A group of symptoms occurring together, indicative of a particular disease or abnormality is known as a ____________________

42. A condition that is a complication of hypocalcemia, and is characterized by severe cramping and twitching of the muscles, and sharp flexion of the wrist and ankle joints is known as ____________________

43. Blood tests that measure the amount of glucose in the blood at the time the sample was drawn are known as ____________________

44. An examination that determines the position, size, shape, and physiological function of the thyroid gland through the use of radionuclear scanning is known as a ____________________

45. The term for an excessive amount of insulin in the body is ____________________

46. The study of the diseases and disorders of the endocrine system is known as ____________________

47. The term for an abnormally low blood calcium level is ____________________

48. The hormone, secreted by the pancreas, that stimulates the liver to convert glycogen to glucose that is then released into the bloodstream is ____________________

49. The breakdown of stored sugar (starch) into simple sugar is known as ____________________

50. Male steroid hormones are also known as ____________________

CHAPTER 13 ALTERNATE COMPLETION QUESTIONS

Emphasizing Word Elements and Abbreviations

(Can be substituted for Completion Questions 36-50)

COMPLETION

INSTRUCTIONS: Read each statement carefully and complete the statement with the most appropriate response. Enter your answer in the space provided.

36. The combining form **acr/o** means ____________

37. The combining form **aden/o** means ____________

38. The combining form **calc/o** means ____________

39. The combining form **cortic/o** means ____________

40. The combining form **crin/o and suffix -crine** mean ____________

41. The combining form **dips/o** means ____________

42. The combining form **kal/i** means ____________

43. The combining form **natr/o** means ____________

44. The combining form for **sweet, sugar** is ____________

45. The combining form for **poisons** is ____________

46. The abbreviation for **fasting blood sugar** is ____________

47. The abbreviation for **adrenocorticotropic hormone** is ____________

48. The abbreviation for **insulin-dependent diabetes mellitus** is ____________

49. The abbreviation for **potassium** is ____________

50. The abbreviation for **sodium** is ____________

CHAPTER 14 SPECIAL SENSES CHAPTER EXAM

MULTIPLE CHOICE

INSTRUCTIONS: The following questions or incomplete statements are followed by four answers or completions. Read each question carefully and select the most appropriate response.

1. Inflammation of the eyelid margins, characterized by redness, swelling, burning, and itching of the margin of the eyelid is known as
   a. astigmatism
   b. blepharitis
   c. presbyopia
   d. blepharoptosis
2. Drooping of the eyelid that partially or entirely covers the eye as a result of a weakened muscle is known as
   a. blepharoptosis
   b. blepharitis
   c. presbyopia
   d. blepharoscopy
3. The lens in the eye becomes progressively cloudy losing its normal transparency and thus altering the perception of images due to the interference of light transmission to the retina is known as a(n)
   a. chalazion
   b. pterygium
   c. cataract
   d. hordeolum
4. Inflammation of the mucous membrane lining the eyelids and covering the front part of the eyeball is known as
   a. chalazion
   b. hordeolum
   c. corneal abrasion
   d. conjunctivitis
5. "Turning out" or eversion of the eyelash margins (especially the lower eyelid) from the eyeball leading to exposure of the eyelid and eyeball surface and lining is known as
   a. ectropion
   b. entropion
   c. esotropia
   d. exotropia
6. An abnormal protrusion of the eyeball(s) is known as
   a. exophthalmia
   b. presbyopia
   c. blepharoptosis
   d. hemianopia
7. Abnormal eyesight in one half of the visual field is known as
   a. glaucoma
   b. hemianopia
   c. exophthalmia
   d. presbyopia
8. An ocular disorder characterized by increase in intraocular pressure is known as
   a. glaucoma
   b. hemianopia
   c. exophthalmia
   d. presbyopia
9. Another name for a stye is
   a. hordeolum
   b. chalazion
   c. exophthalmos
   d. pterygium
10. Another name for farsightedness is
    a. keratitis
    b. hyperopia
    c. myopia
    d. hemianopia
11. Another name for nearsightedness, due to the clarity of close objects, is
    a. keratitis
    b. hyperopia
    c. myopia
    d. hemianopia

12. Vertical, horizontal, rotary, or mixed rhythmic involuntary movements of the eye(s) caused by use of alcohol or certain drugs, lesions on the brain or inner ear, congenital abnormalities, nerve injury at birth, or abnormal retinal development is known as
    a. astigmatism c. chalazion
    b. nystagmus d. strabismus

13. A refractive error occurring after the age of forty, when the lens of the eye(s) cannot focus an image accurately due to its decreasing loss of elasticity resulting in a firmer and more opaque lens is known as
    a. glaucoma c. exophthalmia
    b. hemianopia d. presbyopia

14. An irregular growth developing as a fold in the bulbar conjunctiva on the nasal side of the cornea that can disrupt vision if it extends over the pupil is known as a
    a. hordeolum c. exophthalmos
    b. chalazion d. pterygium

15. Convergent strabismus or "cross-eye" is also known as
    a. ectropion c. esotropia
    b. entropion d. exotropia

16. Divergent strabismus or "wall-eye" is also known as
    a. ectropion c. esotropia
    b. entropion d. exotropia

17. The process of determining the intraocular pressure by calculating the resistance of the eyeball to an applied force causing indentation is known as
    a. tonometry c. keratoplasty
    b. audiometry d. optometry

18. A chronic inner ear disease that is characterized by recurring episodes of vertigo, hearing loss, feeling of pressure or fullness in the affected ear and tinnitus is known as
    a. Meniere's disease c. conductive deafness
    b. serous otitis media d. presbyopia

19. Suppurative otitis, a purulent collection of fluid in the middle ear causing the person to experience pain (possibly severe), an elevation in temperature, dizziness, decreased hearing, vertigo, and tinnitus, is also called
    a. acute otitis media c. otosclerosis
    b. Meniere's disease d. otitis externa

20. The process of measuring how well an individual hears various frequencies of sound waves is known as
    a. otoscopy c. audiometry
    b. otoplasty d. optometry

MATCHING

INSTRUCTIONS: Match the term on the left with the correct definition on the right. Enter your selection in the space provided.

_____ 21. ambiopia	a. inflammation of the lacrimal (tear) gland
_____ 22. blepharospasm	b. one or more spots that appear to drift across the visual field
_____ 23. cycloplegia	c. twitching of the eyelid muscles
_____ 24. dacryoadenitis	d. double vision caused by each eye focusing separately
_____ 25. floaters	e. paralysis of the ciliary muscle of the eye

_____ 26. miotic		a. pain in the ear; earache
_____ 27. mydriatic		b. inflammation of the inner ear
_____ 28. photophobia		c. an agent that causes the pupil of the eye to dilate
_____ 29. labyrinthitis		d. abnormal sensitivity to light, especially by the eyes
_____ 30. otalgia		e. an agent that causes the pupil of the eye to constrict

_____ 31. purulent	a. drainage from the ear; associated with inflammation of the ear
_____ 32. myringoplasty	b. a ringing or tinkling noise heard in the ears
_____ 33. otorrhea	c. surgical incision into the eardrum
_____ 34. tinnitus	d. containing pus
_____ 35. myringotomy	e. surgical repair of the eardrum

COMPLETION

INSTRUCTIONS: Read each statement carefully and complete the statement with the most appropriate response. Enter your answer in the space provided.

36. Any disease of the retina is known as ______________________________

37. The medical term that means pertaining to sound or hearing is ______________________________

38. A recording of the faintest sounds an individual is able to hear is known as an ______________________________

39. Inflammation of one of the mastoid processes of the temporal bone is known as ______________________________

40. Inflammation of the middle ear is known as ______________________________

41. Loss of hearing due to the natural aging process is known as ______________________________

42. A tympanoplasty is the same thing as a ______________________________

43. A sensation of spinning around or of having things in the room or area spinning around the person; a result of disturbance of the equilibrium is known as ______________________________

44. Infection or inflammation of the inner ear is known as ______________________________

45. Inflammation of the outer or external ear canal, called otitis externa, is also known as ______________________________

46. A condition in which the footplate of the stapes becomes immobile and secured to the oval window, resulting in a hearing loss is ______________________________

47. The use of an otoscope to view and examine the tympanic membrane and various parts of the outer ear is known as ______________________________

48. A surgical repair of the ear, in which there is removal of a portion of ear cartilage in order to bring the pinna and auricle nearer the head is a ______________________________

49. A physician who specializes in the study of the diseases and disorders of the eye is known as a(n) ______________________________

50. The instrument used to examine the eyes is a(n) ______________________________

CHAPTER 14 ALTERNATE COMPLETION QUESTIONS

Emphasizing Word Elements and Abbreviations

(Can be substituted for Completion Questions 36-50)

COMPLETION

INSTRUCTIONS: Read each statement carefully and complete the statement with the most appropriate response. Enter your answer in the space provided.

36. The prefix **ambi-** means ______________________________

37. The combining form **ambly/o** means ______________________________

38. The combining form **cor/o** means ______________________________

39. The combining form **lacrim/o** means ______________________________

40. The suffix for **drooping** is ______________________________

41. The combining form that means **glassy** is ______________________________

42. One of the combining forms for **eardrum** is ______________________________

43. One of the combining forms for **hearing** is ______________________________

44. The abbreviation for **each ear (auris unitas)** is ______________________________

45. The abbreviation for **decibel** is ______________________________

46. The abbreviation for **ears, eyes, nose, and throat** is ______________________________

47. The abbreviation for **bilateral otitis media** is ______________________________

48. The abbreviation for **extraocular movement** is ______________________________

49. The abbreviation for **intraocular pressure** is ______________________________

50. The abbreviation for **right eye (ocular dexter)** is ______________________________

CHAPTER 15 URINARY SYSTEM CHAPTER EXAM

MULTIPLE CHOICE

INSTRUCTIONS: The following questions or incomplete statements are followed by four answers or completions. Read each question carefully and select the most appropriate response.

1. An inflammation of the glomerulus of the kidneys, characterized by proteinuria, hematuria, and decreased urine production is known as
   a. glomerulonephritis c. glomerulopathy
   b. hydronephrosis d. pyelitis
2. Distension of the pelvis and calyces of the kidney caused by urine that cannot flow past an obstruction in a ureter is known as
   a. glomerulonephritis c. glomerulopathy
   b. hydronephrosis d. pyelitis
3. A hereditary disorder of the kidneys in which grape-like, fluid-filled sacs or cysts, replace normal kidney tissue is known as
   a. pyelitis c. cystitis
   b. polycystic kidney d. renal cystica
4. A bacterial infection of the renal pelvis of the kidney is known as
   a. glomerulonephritis c. renal cystica
   b. hydronephrosis d. pyelonephritis
5. An abnormal back flow of urine from the bladder to the ureter is known as
   a. vesicoureteroreflux c. urethritis
   b. ureteropathy d. vesicourethritis
6. The process of removing excess fluids and toxins from the blood by continually shunting the patient's blood from the body into a dialysis machine, for filtering, and then returning the clean blood to the patient's bloodstream is known as
   a. peritoneal dialysis c. continuous cycling peritoneal dialysis
   b. hemodialysis d. arterial catheterization
7. An examination performed to evaluate bladder tone is known as
   a. renography c. cystometrography
   b. cystocele d. vesicotonotomy
8. An x-ray of the lower abdomen that defines the size, shape, and location of the kidneys, ureters, and bladder without the use of a contrast medium is a(n)
   a. renogram c. KUB
   b. pyelogram d. IVP
9. A radiographic procedure in which small-caliber catheters are passed through a cystoscope into the ureters in order to visualize the ureters and the renal pelvis is known as a(n)
   a. intravenous pyelogram c. kidneys, ureters, bladder
   b. retrograde pyelogram d. vesicotonotomy
10. X-ray visualization of the bladder and urethra during the voiding process, after the bladder has been filled with a contrast material is known as a
    a. direct visualization c. vesicoureteroreflux
    b. voiding cystourethrogram d. urinary fluoroscopy

11. The clean-catch urine specimen is also known as a
    a. first-voided specimen
    b. residual specimen
    c. mid-stream specimen
    d. sterile specimen

12. When the patient is instructed to collect a specimen as soon as he or she arises in the morning and to refrigerate it until it can be taken to the medical office or laboratory, he/she is collecting a
    a. sterile specimen
    b. residual specimen
    c. clean-catch specimen
    d. first-voided specimen

13. The central collecting area of the kidney is known as the
    a. renal pelvis
    b. cortex
    c. ureter
    d. urethra

14. The muscular tubes lined with mucous membrane, one leading from each kidney down to the urinary bladder, are known as the
    a. urethras
    b. ureters
    c. calyces
    d. glomeruli

15. The depression, or pit, of the kidney where the vessels and nerves enter is the
    a. fossa
    b. ureter
    c. trigone area
    d. hilum

16. As blood passes through the glomeruli of the kidneys, the blood pressure forces materials through the glomerular walls and into the Bowman's capsule: this process is known as
    a. glomerular filtration
    b. glomerular secretion
    c. glomerular absorption
    d. micturition

17. A substance that inhibits the growth and reproduction of microorganisms is known as a(n)
    a. antiseptic
    b. hemoseptic
    c. hemolysis agent
    d. astringent

18. The cup-shaped end of a renal tubule containing, or surrounding, a glomerulus is known as
    a. the hilum
    b. the fossa
    c. Bowman's capsule
    d. Henle's loop

19. The membrane lining the abdominal cavity is known as the
    a. petechia
    b. peritoneum
    c. visceral pleura
    d. fascia

20. A hormone, produced by the kidneys, that stimulates the production of red blood cells within the bone marrow is
    a. erythropoietin
    b. hemolysin
    c. erythromyelomycin
    d. renin

MATCHING

INSTRUCTIONS: Match the term on the left with the correct definition on the right. Enter your selection in the space provided.

_____ 21. glycosuria	a. urination, especially excessive, at night
_____ 22. hematuria	b. presence of excessive amounts of ketone bodies in the urine
_____ 23. ketonuria	c. secretion of a diminished amount of urine in relation to the fluid intake; scanty urine output
_____ 24. nocturia	d. abnormal presence of a sugar, especially glucose, in the urine
_____ 25. oliguria	e. abnormal presence of blood in the urine

_____ 26. polydipsia	a. a feeling of the need to void urine immediately
_____ 27. polyuria	b. the presence of pus in the urine, usually a sign of an infection of the urinary tract
_____ 28. pyuria	c. excessive thirst
_____ 29. urgency	d. inflammation of the urinary bladder
_____ 30. cystitis	e. excretion of abnormally large amounts of urine

_____ 31. dysuria	a. the act of eliminating urine from the bladder
_____ 32. albuminuria	b. the presence of bacteria in the urine
_____ 33. bacteriuria	c. the cessation (stopping) of urine production
_____ 34. anuria	d. the presence of abnormally large quantities of protein in the urine
_____ 35. micturation	e. painful urination

COMPLETION

INSTRUCTIONS: Read each statement carefully and complete the statement with the most appropriate response. Enter your answer in the space provided.

36. The smallest branch of an artery is a(n) ____________________

37. The cup-shaped end of a renal tubule containing a glomerulus is known as ____________________

38. The outer layer of a body organ or structure is the ____________________

39. An instrument used to view the interior of the bladder, ureter, or kidney is a ____________________

40. The solution that contains water and electrolytes that passes through the artificial kidney to remove excess fluids and wastes from the blood is called the ____________________

41. The process of removing waste products from the blood when the kidneys are unable to do so is known as ____________________

42. The length of time the dialysis solution stays in the peritoneal cavity during peritoneal dialysis is known as ____________________

43. A ball-shaped collection of very tiny, coiled and intertwined capillaries, located in the cortex of the kidney is known as the ____________________

44. The most internal part of a structure or organ is the ____________________

45. Another name for kidney stones or renal calculi is ____________________

46. Inflammation of the membrane lining the abdominal cavity is known as ____________________

47. Urine that remains in the bladder after urination is called ____________________

48. Urine that is said to be turbid will appear ____________________

49. The presence of excessive amounts of urea and other nitrogenous waste products in the blood is known as ____________________

50. The inability to control urination is known as ____________________

CHAPTER 15 ALTERNATE COMPLETION QUESTIONS

Emphasizing Word Elements and Abbreviations

(Can be substituted for Completion Questions 36-50)

COMPLETION

INSTRUCTIONS: Read each statement carefully and complete the statement with the most appropriate response. Enter your answer in the space provided.

36. The combining form **azot/o** means ________________________

37. The combining form **cali/o or calic/o** means ________________________

38. The combining form **nephr/o** means ________________________

39. The combining form **olig/o** means ________________________

40. The combining form **pyel/o** means ________________________

41. The abbreviation **CCPD** means ________________________

42. The abbreviation **ESRD** means ________________________

43. The abbreviation **IVP** means ________________________

44. The abbreviation for the **degree of acidity or alkalinity of a solution** is ________________________

45. The abbreviation **UTI** means ________________________

46. The combining form **py/o** means ________________________

47. One combining form for **urinary bladder** is ________________________

48. The suffix that means **urine condition** is ________________________

49. One combining form for **ketone bodies** is ________________________

50. The combining form for **meatus** is ________________________

CHAPTER 16 MALE REPRODUCTIVE SYSTEM CHAPTER EXAM

MULTIPLE CHOICE

INSTRUCTIONS: The following questions or incomplete statements are followed by four answers or completions. Read each question carefully and select the most appropriate response.

1. The absence of one or both testicles is known as
   a. anorchism
   b. balanitis
   c. cryptorchidism
   d. testiculitis
2. Inflammation of the glans penis and the mucous membrane beneath it is known as
   a. anorchism
   b. balanitis
   c. cryptorchidism
   d. testiculitis
3. A benign enlargement of the prostate gland, creating pressure on the upper part of the urethra or neck of the bladder, causing obstruction to the flow of urine is known as
   a. testiculitis
   b. benign prostatic hypotrophy
   c. benign cryptorchidism
   d. benign prostatic hypertrophy
4. A condition of undescended testicle(s) is known as
   a. anorchism
   b. balanitis
   c. cryptorchidism
   d. testiculitis
5. A congenital defect in which the urethra opens on the upper side of the penis at some point near the glans is called
   a. hydrocele
   b. epispadias
   c. anorchism
   d. hypospadias
6. An accumulation of fluid in any sac-like cavity or duct, particularly the scrotal sac or along the spermatic cord is known as
   a. hydrocele
   b. epispadias
   c. anorchism
   d. hypospadias
7. A congenital defect in which the urethra opens on the underside of the penis instead of at the end is known as
   a. hydrocele
   b. epispadias
   c. anorchism
   d. hypospadias
8. A protrusion of a part of the intestine through a weakened spot in the muscles and membranes of the inguinal region of the abdomen is known as a(n)
   a. inguinal hernia
   b. umbilical hernia
   c. inguinal fistula
   d. lumbosacral hernia
9. A tightness of the foreskin (prepuce) of the penis that prevents it from being pulled back, creating a narrowed opening of the foreskin, is known as
   a. prostatitis
   b. balanitis
   c. phimosis
   d. hypospadias
10. An abnormal dilation of the veins of the spermatic cord leading to the testicle is known as
    a. phimosis
    b. varicocele
    c. inguinal hernia
    d. spermatic dilations

11. Genital herpes differs from other sexually transmitted diseases in that
    a. it disappears without treatment within six weeks
    b. it affects only men
    c. it can recur spontaneously once the virus has been acquired
    d. it is accompanied by a purplish-red rash on the trunk of the body

12. A surgical procedure in which the foreskin (prepuce) of the penis is removed is called a(n)
    a. circumcision
    b. epididymectomy
    c. balanectomy
    d. orchidoplasty

13. The surgical removal of the prostate gland by making an incision into the abdominal wall, just above the pubis is known as a
    a. retrograde pyelogram
    b. transurethral prostatectomy
    c. laparoscopy
    d. suprapubic prostatectomy

14. The surgical removal of the prostate gland by inserting a resectoscope through the urethra and into the bladder to remove small pieces of tissue from the prostate gland is known as a
    a. retrograde pyelogram
    b. transurethral prostatectomy
    c. laparoscopy
    d. suprapubic prostatectomy

15. The medical term for a male sterilization is a
    a. vasectomy
    b. epididymectomy
    c. orchiopexy
    d. balanectomy

16. A skin lesion, usually of primary syphilis, that begins at the site of infection as a small raised area and develops into a red, painless ulcer with a scooped-out appearance is called a(n)
    a. scar
    b. chancre
    c. fissure
    d. ulcer

17. A loose, retractable fold of skin covering the tip of the penis, the foreskin, is also called the
    a. prepuce
    b. ectoderm
    c. cortex
    d. perineum

18. Surgical repair of the glans penis is called a(n)
    a. orchiectomy
    b. laparoscopy
    c. balanoplasty
    d. cryosurgery

19. The area between the scrotum and the anus in the male is known as the
    a. perineum
    b. prepuce
    c. peritoneum
    d. sigmoid colon

20. The male gonads, or male sex glands that are responsible for production of spermatozoa, and for the secretion of the male hormone, testosterone are called the
    a. seminiferous tubules
    b. bulbourethral glands
    c. vas deferens
    d. testicles

MATCHING

INSTRUCTIONS: Match the term on the left with the correct definition on the right. Enter your selection in the space provided.

_____ 21. anorexia
_____ 22. asymptomatic
_____ 23. cryosurgery
_____ 24. debridement
_____ 25. dormant

a. the removal of dirt, damaged tissue, and cellular debris from a wound or a burn to prevent infection and to promote healing
b. inactive
c. without symptoms
d. use of subfreezing temperature to destroy tissue
e. loss of appetite

______	26. dysuria	a. the tip of the penis
______	27. ejaculation	b. the male sex glands that are called the testes
______	28. epididymis	c. painful urination
______	29. gonad	d. the process of expelling semen from the male urethra
______	30. glans penis	e. a tightly coiled tubule, resembling a comma, that houses the sperm until they mature

______	31. malaise	a. a gland that surrounds the base of the urethra that secretes a milky colored secretion into the urethra during ejaculation
______	32. malodorous	b. removal of the prostate gland
______	33. palpation	c. foul smelling; having a bad odor
______	34. prostate gland	d. a technique used in physical examinations that involves feeling parts of the body with the hands
______	35. prostatectomy	e. a vague feeling of bodily weakness or discomfort, often marking the onset of disease

COMPLETION

INSTRUCTIONS: Read each statement carefully and complete the statement with the most appropriate response. Enter your answer in the space provided.

36. Inflammation of the epididymis is known as ______________________________

37. A malignant growth that begins as soft, brownish or purple raised areas on the feet and slowly spreads in the skin, spreading to the lymph nodes and internal organs, that occurs most often in men and is associated with AIDS is known as ______________________________

38. Any agent or regimen that contributes to the prevention of infection and disease is known as a ______________________________

39. An instrument used to view the rectum, that has a cutting and cauterizing (burning) loop is called a ______________________________

40. An instrument used to surgically remove tissue from the body, that has a light source and lens attached for viewing the area, is known as a ______________________________

41. Urine that remains in the bladder after urination is called ______________________________

42. An external sac that houses the testicles; located posterior to the penis and is suspended from the perineum is known as the ______________________________

43. A combination of sperm and various secretions that is expelled from the body, through the urethra, during sexual intercourse is called ________________

44. Specialized coils of tiny tubules that are responsible for production of sperm, located in the testes, are known as the ________________

45. A mature male germ cell is a ________________

46. A male hormone, secreted by the testes, that is responsible for the secondary sex characteristic changes that occur in the male with the onset of puberty, is ________________

47. A small tubular structure, extending the length of the penis, that transports urine from the bladder and the semen, when ejaculated, to the outside of the body is the ________________

48. The narrow, straight tube that transports sperm from the epididymis to the ejaculatory duct is the ________________

49. Another name for blisters is ________________

50. A surgical cutting and tying of the vas deferens to prevent the passage of sperm, consequently preventing pregnancy, is called a ________________

CHAPTER 16 ALTERNATE COMPLETION QUESTIONS
Emphasizing Word Elements and Abbreviations

(Can be substituted for Completion Questions 36-50)

COMPLETION

INSTRUCTIONS: Read each statement carefully and complete the statement with the most appropriate response. Enter your answer in the space provided.

36. The combining form **andr/o** means ____________________

37. The combining form **crypt/o** means ____________________

38. The combining form **orchi/o** means ____________________

39. The combining form **semin/i** means ____________________

40. The combining form for **glans penis** is ____________________

41. The abbreviation for **benign prostatic hypertrophy** is ____________________

42. The abbreviation for **gonorrhea** is ____________________

43. The abbreviation for **intravenous pyelogram** is ____________________

44. The abbreviation for **serological test for syphilis** is ____________________

45. The abbreviation for **transurethral resection of the prostate gland** is ____________________

46. The combining form **test/o** means ____________________

47. The combining form that means **cold** is ____________________

48. The combining form that means **prostate gland** is ____________________

49. The combining form that means **animal (man)** is ____________________

50. The combining form **spermat/o** means ____________________

CHAPTER 17 FEMALE REPRODUCTIVE SYSTEM CHAPTER EXAM

MULTIPLE CHOICE

INSTRUCTIONS: The following questions or incomplete statements are followed by four answers or completions. Read each question carefully and select the most appropriate response.

1. An acute or chronic inflammation of the uterine cervix is known as
   a. cervicitis c. endometrial carcinoma
   b. a cystocele d. cervicectomy

2. A herniation or downward protrusion of the urinary bladder through the wall of the vagina is known as a(n)
   a. uterine polyp c. cystocele
   b. fibroid tumor d. adenexa

3. A malignant tumor of the inner lining of the uterus is known as
   a. adenocystocele c. uterine sarcoidosis
   b. endometrial carcinoma d. fibroid tumor

4. The presence and growth of endometrial tissue in areas outside the lining of the uterus is known as
   a. endometriosis c. fibroid tumors
   b. adenocystocele d. endometrial carcinoma

5. The presence of single or multiple fluid-filled cysts that are palpable in the breasts, and that fluctuate in size with the menstrual period, becoming tender just before menstruation, is known as
   a. ovarian carcinoma c. fibrocystic breast disease
   b. mastitis d. adenocarcinoma of the breast

6. Another name for pelvic inflammatory disease is
   a. salpingitis c. fallopianitis
   b. pelvicitis d. endometriosis

7. An invasive procedure in which a needle is inserted into an area of the body, such as the breast, to withdraw a tissue or fluid sample for microscopic examination and diagnosis is known as a(n)
   a. aspiration biopsy c. conization
   b. mastectomy d. lumpectomy

8. Visual examination of the vagina and cervix using an instrument with a lighted binocular microscope for direct examination of the surfaces of the vagina and cervix is known as a(n)
   a. conization c. colposcopy
   b. pelvimetry d. laparoscopy

9. Surgical removal of a cone-shaped segment of the cervix for diagnosis or treatment is known as a(n)
   a. conization c. colpectomy
   b. pelvimetry d. laparotomy

10. The destruction of tissue by rapid freezing with substances such as liquid nitrogen is known as
    a. electrocauterization c. conization
    b. cryosurgery d. fluoroscopy

11. The surgical puncture through the posterior wall of the vagina into the cul-de-sac to withdraw intraperitoneal fluid for examination is known as a(n)
    a. colposcopy c. laparotomy
    b. culdocentesis d. vaginal biopsy

12. Dilatation or widening of the cervical canal with a dilator, followed by scraping of the uterine lining with a curet is known as a(n)
    a. dilatation and curettage
    b. conization
    c. hysterosalpingography
    d. pap smear

13. The process of x-raying the soft tissue of the breast, for the purpose of detecting various benign and/or malignant growths before they can be felt is called
    a. mammography
    b. hysterosalpingography
    c. mammometry
    d. breast fluoroscopy

14. A microscopic examination of cells scraped from within the cervix (endocervix), from around the cervix (ectocervix), and from the posterior part of the vagina (near the cervix) to test for cervical cancer is known as a
    a. culdocentesis
    b. endometrial biopsy
    c. conization
    d. pap smear

15. The darker pigmented, circular area surrounding the nipple of each breast is known as the
    a. alveoli
    b. areola
    c. papillae
    d. adnexa

16. The neck of the uterus is also known as the
    a. adnexa
    b. cervix
    c. fallopian tube
    d. oviduct

17. The cessation of menstruation, or menopause, is known as the
    a. climacteric
    b. menarche
    c. climax
    d. fourchette

18. Which of the following medical terms means the same as sexual intercourse
    1. clitoris
    2. coitus
    3. copulation
    4. fertilization

    a. 1, 4
    b. 1, 3
    c. 2, 3
    d. 3, 4

19. A yellowish mass that forms within the ruptured ovarian follicle after ovulation and functions as a temporary endocrine gland for the purpose of secreting estrogen and large amounts of progesterone that will sustain pregnancy, should it occur, until the placenta forms, is known as the
    a. corpus luteum
    b. cul-de-sac
    c. fallopian fimbriae
    d. endometrium

20. The dome-shaped central, upper portion of the uterus between the points of insertion of the fallopian tubes is known as the
    a. cul-de-sac
    b. fourchette
    c. fundus
    d. hymen

MATCHING

INSTRUCTIONS: Match the term on the left with the correct definition on the right. Enter your selection in the space provided.

_____ 21. amenorrhea
_____ 22. dysmenorrhea
_____ 23. menorrhagia
_____ 24. metrorrhagia
_____ 25. oligomenorrhea

a. painful menstrual flow
b. abnormally long or very heavy menstrual periods
c. abnormally light or infrequent menstruation
d. absence of menstrual flow
e. uterine bleeding at times other than the menstrual period

_____ 26. cervix
_____ 27. endometrium
_____ 28. fertilization
_____ 29. fimbriae
_____ 30. fourchette

a. the fringelike end of the fallopian tube
b. inner lining of the uterus
c. the point on the posterior rim of the vaginal opening at which the labia minora connect
d. the neck of the uterus
e. the union of a male sperm and a female ovum

_____ 31. gamete
_____ 32. gonads
_____ 33. hymen
_____ 34. labia majora
_____ 35. mammary glands

a. gamete-producing glands, such as the ovaries or testes
b. two folds of skin containing fatty tissue and covered with hair that lie on either side of the vaginal opening, extending from the mons pubis to the perineum
c. the female breasts
d. a mature sperm or ovum
e. a thin layer of elastic, connective tissue membrane that forms a border around the outer opening of the vagina and may partially cover the vaginal opening

COMPLETION

INSTRUCTIONS: Read each statement carefully and complete the statement with the most appropriate response. Enter your answer in the space provided.

36. The onset of menstruation, or first menstrual period is called the ____________________

37. The permanent cessation (stopping) of the menstrual cycles is known as ____________________

38. The periodic shedding of the lining of the nonpregnant uterus through a bloody discharge, that passes through the vagina to the outside of the body, and occurs at monthly intervals that last for 3-5 days, is known as ____________________

39. The muscular layer of the wall of the uterus is known as the ____________________

40. One of a pair of female gonads responsible for producing mature ova and releasing them during ovulation, also responsible for producing the female hormones estrogen and progesterone, is known as a(n) ____________________

41. The female reproductive cell, or female sex cell, is known as the ____________________

42. The area between the vaginal orifice and the anus that is composed of muscular and fibrous tissue and serves as support for the pelvic structures is known as the ____________________

43. The period of intrauterine development of the fetus from conception through birth is known as ____________________

44. A group of symptoms that include irritability, fluid retention, tenderness of the breasts, and a general feeling of depression, occurring shortly before the onset of menstruation is called ____________________ ____________________

45. The period of life at which the ability to reproduce begins; i.e., in the female, it is the period when the female reproductive organs are fully developed and is called ____________________

46. A mature male germ cell is called a ____________________

47. The hollow, pear-shaped organ of the female reproductive system that houses the fertilized, implanted ovum as it develops throughout pregnancy is the ____________________

48. The muscular tube that connects the uterus with the vulva is the ____________________

49. The female external genitalia that consists of the mons pubis, labia majora, clitoris, labia minora, vestibule, urinary meatus, vaginal orifice, Bartholin's glands, and the perineum is collectively referred to as the ____________________

50. Surgically cutting and tying the fallopian tubes to prevent passage of ova or sperm through the tubes, consequently preventing pregnancy, is known as a ____________________

CHAPTER 17 ALTERNATE COMPLETION QUESTIONS

Emphasizing Word Elements and Abbreviations

(Can be substituted for Completion Questions 36-50)

COMPLETION

INSTRUCTIONS: Read each statement carefully and complete the statement with the most appropriate response. Enter your answer in the space provided.

36. The prefix **ante-** means ______________________________

37. The suffix **-arche** means ______________________________

38. The combining form **colp/o** means ______________________________

39. The combining form **mamm/o** means ______________________________

40. The combining form for **menstruation** is ______________________________

41. One combining form for **uterus** is ______________________________

42. One combining form for **ovary** is ______________________________

43. The combining form for **fallopian tubes** is ______________________________

44. The suffix that means **discharge or flow** is ______________________________

45. The abbreviation for **dilation and curettage** is ______________________________

46. The abbreviation for **endometrial biopsy** is ______________________________

47. The abbreviation for **gynecology** is ______________________________

48. The abbreviation for **last menstrual period** is ______________________________

49. The abbreviation for **pelvic inflammatory disease** is ______________________________

50. The abbreviation for **premenstrual syndrome** is ______________________________

CHAPTER 18 OBSTETRICS CHAPTER EXAM

MULTIPLE CHOICE

INSTRUCTIONS: The following questions or incomplete statements are followed by four answers or completions. Read each question carefully and select the most appropriate response.

1. The settling of the fetal head into the pelvis, occurring a few weeks prior to the onset of labor is known as
   a. lightening
   b. quickening
   c. Hegar's sign
   d. ballottment
2. A darkened vertical midline appearing on the abdomen of a pregnant woman, extending from the fundus to the symphysis pubis, is called
   a. chloasma
   b. linea nigra
   c. striae
   d. quickening
3. A position in which the patient lies upon her back, buttocks even with the end of the table, with her knees bent back toward her abdomen and the heel of each foot resting in an elevated foot rest at the end of the exam table, is called
   a. lithotomy position
   b. trendelenburg position
   c. knee-chest position
   d. Sim's position
4. A woman who has been pregnant more than once is known as a(n)
   a. primigravida
   b. nulligravida
   c. multigravida
   d. multipara
5. A formula that is used to calculate the date of birth; subtracting 3 months from the first day of the last normal menstrual period and adding 7 days to that date to arrive at the estimated date of birth, is called
   a. Nagele's rule
   b. Goodell's rule
   c. Hager's rule
   d. Chadwick's rule
6. The release of the mature ovum from the ovary; occurs approximately 14 days prior to the beginning of menses is termed
   a. menarche
   b. ovulation
   c. quickening
   d. parturition
7. A woman who has given birth for the first time, after a pregnancy of at least 20 weeks gestation, is known as a(n)
   a. primigravida
   b. primipara
   c. nulligravida
   d. nullipara
8. The first feeling of movement of the fetus felt by the expectant mother, usually occurring around 18-20 weeks' gestation, is known as
   a. ballottment
   b. Hegar's sign
   c. Goodell's sign
   d. quickening
9. Stretch marks that occur during pregnancy due to the great amount of stretching that occurs are called
   a. striae gravidarum
   b. chloasma
   c. linea nigra
   d. varicosities
10. One of the three periods of approximately 3 months into which pregnancy is divided is known as a(n)
    a. trimester
    b. quarter
    c. one lunar month
    d. gestational segment

11. As pregnancy progresses women usually display a manner of walking in which the feet are wide apart and the walk resembles that of a duck. This is called a
    a. pregnant stride
    b. waddling gait
    c. shuffling gait
    d. lordotic gait

12. Termination of a pregnancy before the fetus has reached a viable age, i.e., an age at which the fetus could live outside of the uterine environment is known as a(n)
    a. ectopic pregnancy
    b. abruptio placenta
    c. abortion
    d. placenta previa

13. The premature separation of a normally implanted placenta from the uterine wall, after the pregnancy has passed 20 weeks gestation or during labor, is known as
    a. ectopic pregnancy
    b. abruptio placenta
    c. abortion
    d. placenta previa

14. Abnormal implantation of a fertilized ovum outside of the uterine cavity is called a(n)
    a. embryo
    b. Rh incompatibility
    c. hydatidiform mole
    d. ectopic pregnancy

15. Women who are not diabetic before pregnancy, and develop an inability to metabolize carbohydrates (glucose intolerance), with resultant hyperglycemia, have a condition known as
    a. gestational diabetes
    b. diabetes insipidus
    c. juvenile diabetes
    d. hyperemesis gravidarum

16. An abnormal condition of pregnancy characterized by severe vomiting that results in maternal dehydration, and weight loss, is known as
    a. gestational diabetes
    b. hyperemesis gravidarum
    c. hydatidiform mole
    d. placenta previa

17. A condition in which the cervical os dilates before the fetus reaches term, without labor or uterine contractions, is known as a(n)
    a. incompetent cervix
    b. cerclage
    c. placenta previa
    d. abruptio placenta

18. A stress test used to evaluate the ability of the fetus to tolerate the stress of labor and delivery, is known as a
    a. tread mill test
    b. fetal monitor
    c. contraction stress test
    d. pelvimetry

19. The process of measuring the female pelvis, manually or by x-ray, to determine its adequacy for childbearing, is known as a
    a. tread mill test
    b. fetal monitor
    c. contraction stress test
    d. pelvimetry

20. Testing that is performed on maternal urine and/or blood to determine the presence of the hormone HCG (human chorionic gonadotropin), is a test performed to confirm
    a. menarche
    b. pregnancy
    c. menopause
    d. a ruptured amniotic sac

MATCHING

INSTRUCTIONS: Match the term on the left with the correct definition on the right. Enter your selection in the space provided.

_____ 21. amenorrhea
_____ 22. amniotic sac
_____ 23. areola
_____ 24. ballottement
_____ 25. Braxton-Hick's contractions

a. the double-layered sac that contains the fetus and the amniotic fluid during pregnancy
b. the darker pigmented, circular area surrounding the nipple of each breast
c. irregular, ineffective, contractions of the uterus that occur throughout pregnancy
d. absence of menstrual flow
e. A technique of using the examiner's finger to tap against the uterus, through the vagina, to cause the fetus to "bounce' within the amniotic fluid and feeling it rebound quickly

_____ 26. cerclage
_____ 27. cesarean section
_____ 28. Chadwick's sign
_____ 29. chloasma
_____ 30. chorion

a. the outer of the two membrane layers that surround and contain the fetus and the amniotic fluid during pregnancy
b. suturing the cervix to keep it from dilating prematurely during the pregnancy
c. patches of tan or brown pigmentation associated with pregnancy, occurring mostly on the forehead, cheeks, and nose
d. the bluish-violet hue of the cervix and vagina after approximately the 6th week of pregnancy
e. a surgical procedure in which the abdomen and uterus are incised and a baby is delivered transabdominally

_____ 31. coitus
_____ 32. colostrum
_____ 33. conception
_____ 34. corpus luteum
_____ 35. eclampsia

a. the most severe form of hypertension during pregnancy, evidenced by seizures
b. a mass of yellowish tissue that forms in the ruptured ovarian follicle after ovulation
c. sexual intercourse
d. thin, yellowish fluid secreted by breasts during pregnancy and the first few days after birth, before lactation begins
e. the union of a male sperm and a female ovum

COMPLETION

INSTRUCTIONS: Read each statement carefully and complete the statement with the most appropriate response. Enter your answer in the space provided.

36. Swelling of the tissues with water retention is known as ______________________________

37. Thinning of the cervix that allows it to enlarge the diameter of its opening in preparation for childbirth is known as ______________________________

38. The inner lining of the uterus is known as the ______________________________

39. A surgical procedure in which an incision is made into the woman's perineum to enlarge the vaginal opening for delivery of the baby is called a(n) ______________________________

40. A special stethoscope for hearing the fetal heartbeat through the mother's abdomen is known as a(n) ______________________________

41. The name given to the developing baby from approximately the 8th week after conception until birth (about the 3rd month) is a(n) ______________________________

42. The superior aspect of the uterus is called the ______________________________

43. A mature sperm or ovum is called a ______________________________

44. The term of pregnancy that equals approximately 280 days from the onset of the last menstrual period is known as ______________________________

45. The softening of the uterine cervix, a probable sign of pregnancy is called ______________

46. A woman who is pregnant is known as a ______________________________

47. Softening of the lower segment of the uterus; a probable sign of pregnancy, is known as ______________________________

48. The time and the processes that occur during the process of giving birth, from the beginning of cervical dilatation to the delivery of the placenta is known as ______________________________

49. The production and secretion of milk from the female breasts as nourishment for the infant, is known as ______________________________

50. Visualization of the abdominal cavity with an instrument called a laparoscope, through an incision into the abdominal wall is called a(n) ______________________________

CHAPTER 18 ALTERNATE COMPLETION QUESTIONS
Emphasizing Word Elements and Abbreviations

(Can be substituted for Completion Questions 36-50)

COMPLETION

INSTRUCTIONS: Read each statement carefully and complete the statement with the most appropriate response. Enter your answer in the space provided.

36. The combining form **amni/o** means ______________________________

37. The combining form **culd/o** means ______________________________

38. The combining form **episi/o** means ______________________________

39. The combining form **fet/o** means ______________________________

40. The suffix **-gravida** means ______________________________

41. The combining form **lact/o** means ______________________________

42. The prefix **multi-** means ______________________________

43. The suffix that means **to give birth** is ______________________________

44. The prefix that means **first** is ______________________________

45. The combining form that means **midwife** is ______________________________

46. The abbreviation for **expected date of delivery** is ______________________________

47. The abbreviation for **fetal heart rate** is ______________________________

48. The abbreviation for **pregnant** is ______________________________

49. The abbreviation **LMP** means ______________________________

50. The abbreviation **NSD** means ______________________________

CHAPTER 19 CHILD HEALTH CHAPTER EXAM

MULTIPLE CHOICE

INSTRUCTIONS: The following questions or incomplete statements are followed by four answers or completions. Read each question carefully and select the most appropriate response.

1. A viral disease characterized by sudden onset with slight fever, successive eruptions of macules, papules, and vesicles on the skin, followed by crusting over of the lesions with a granular scab, is known as
   a. chickenpox
   b. rubella
   c. rubeola
   d. scarlatina

2. A viral disease characterized by a fiery red rash on the cheeks, giving the face the appearance of "slapped cheeks", is known as
   a. rubella
   b. rubeola
   c. scarlatina
   d. fifth disease

3. A contagious, superficial, staphylococcal/streptococcal skin infection characterized by serous vesicles and pustules that form crusted-over lesions, usually forming on the face, is known as
   a. scarlatina
   b. impetigo
   c. fifth disease
   d. scabies

4. Another name for mumps is
   a. impetigo
   b. erythema infectiosum
   c. infectious parotitis
   d. fifth disease

5. Another name for pertussis is
   a. whooping cough
   b. measles
   c. mumps
   d. fifth disease

6. Rubella is also known as
   1. German measles
   2. red measles
   3. three-day measles
   4. roseola

   a. 1, 3, 4
   b. 1, 3
   c. 2, 4
   d. 1, 2, 3

7. An acute, highly communicable viral disease, lasting 7-10 days, that is characterized by a typical red, blotchy rash beginning behind the ears, on the forehead or cheeks, and progressing to the extremities and trunk, is known as
   a. rubeola
   b. rubella
   c. scarlatina
   d. roseola

8. An acute, contagious disease characterized by a sore throat, abrupt high fever, a "strawberry" tongue (red and swollen), and a pointlike bright red rash on the body is known as
   a. rubeola
   b. rubella
   c. scarlatina
   d. roseola

9. A respiratory disorder characterized by paroxysmal dyspnea, accompanied by wheezing caused by a spasm of the bronchial tubes, with attacks lasting from 30 minutes to several hours, is known as
   a. emphysema
   b. asthma
   c. croup
   d. diphtheria

10. A congenital defect in which there is an open space between the nasal cavity and the lip, due to failure of the soft tissue and bones in this area to fuse properly during embryologic development, is known as a
    a. cleft lip
    b. cleft palate
    c. nasopharyngeal anomaly
    d. coarctated lip

11. A childhood disease characterized by a barking cough, suffocative and difficult breathing, stridor, and laryngeal spasm is known as
    a. emphysema
    b. asthma
    c. croup
    d. impetigo

12. A condition of undescended testicles is known as
    a. cryptorchidism
    b. cryptorchiectomy
    c. cryptosis
    d. orchidism

13. Generalized growth retardation of the body due to the deficiency of the human growth hormone, before puberty, is known as
    a. dwarfism
    b. gigantism
    c. hyperpituitarism
    d. trisomy 21

14. A congenital defect in which the urethra opens on the upper side of the penis at some point near the glans is known as
    a. hyperpituitarism
    b. hypospadias
    c. epispadias
    d. phimosis

15. A proportional overgrowth of the body's tissue due to hypersecretion of the human growth hormone before puberty is known as
    a. dwarfism
    b. gigantism
    c. hyperpituitarism
    d. trisomy 21

16. Respiratory distress syndrome of the premature infant (RDS) is also known as
    a. hyaline membrane disease
    b. trisomy 21
    c. diphtheria
    d. Reye's syndrome

17. An accumulation of fluid in the scrotal sac or along the spermatic cord is known as a(n)
    a. hemorrhoid
    b. hydrocele
    c. sclerotic cordi
    d. ascites

18. A congenital defect in which the urethra opens on the underside of the penis instead of at the end is known as
    a. hyperpituitarism
    b. hypospadias
    c. epispadias
    d. phimosis

19. A tightness of the foreskin of the penis of the male infant, that prevents it from being pulled back, is known as
    a. patent ductus urethrosis
    b. epispadias
    c. phimosis
    d. cryptorchidism

20. The completely unexpected and unexplained death of an apparently well infant is called "crib death"; this condition is also known as
    a. Tay-Sachs disease
    b. sudden infant death syndrome
    c. fifth disease
    d. Reye's syndrome

MATCHING

INSTRUCTIONS: Match the term on the left with the correct definition on the right. Enter your selection in the space provided.

_____ 21. active immunity
_____ 22. immunization
_____ 23. natural immunity
_____ 24. vaccine
_____ 25. toxoid

a. an innate and permanent form of immunity to a specific disease
b. a toxin that has been treated with chemicals or with heat to decrease its toxic effect but that retains its antigenic power
c. immunity acquired as a result of disease or immunization
d. a process by which resistance to an infectious disease is induced or augmented
e. a suspension of attenuated or killed microorganisms

_____ 26. apnea
_____ 27. crackles
_____ 28. friction rub
_____ 29. grunting
_____ 30. stridor

a. absence of respirations
b. abnormal, short audible gruntlike breaks in exhalation that often accompany severe chest pain
c. an abnormal, high-pitched, musical sound, caused by an obstruction in the trachea or larynx
d. a common abnormal respiratory sound heard on auscultation of the chest during inspiration, characterized by discontinuous bubbling noises
e. a dry, grating sound heard with a stethoscope during auscultation

_____ 31. stature
_____ 32. congenital
_____ 33. pyrexia
_____ 34. cyanosis
_____ 35. omphalorrhea

a. present at birth
b. bluish discoloration of the skin and mucous membranes
c. drainage from the umbilicus
d. fever
e. natural height of a person in an upright position

COMPLETION

INSTRUCTIONS: Read each statement carefully and complete the statement with the most appropriate response. Enter your answer in the space provided.

36. The number of primary teeth erupting between the ages of 6 to 30 months of age is ____________

37. An increase in the whole or any of its parts physically is known as ____________

38. The measurement of the distance from the crown of the infant's head to the infant's heel, while the infant is lying on his/her back with legs extended, is a measurement of ____________

39. The introduction of a hollow needle and stylet into the subarachnoid space of the lumbar portion of the spinal canal, for the purpose of withdrawing cerebrospinal fluid, is known as a(n) ____________

40. A congenital anomaly characterized by abnormal smallness of the head in relation to the rest of the body and by underdevelopment of the brain, is known as ______________________________

41. The medical specialty concerned with the diseases and abnormalities of the newborn infant is known as ______________________________

42. An inflammation of the umbilical stump, marked by redness, swelling, and purulent exudate in severe cases, is known as ______________________________

43. The body temperature as measured electronically at the eardrum is known as a ______________________________

44. The mean body temperature of a normal person as recorded by a clinical thermometer placed in the mouth is known as a(n) ______________________________

45. A physician who specializes in the preventive and primary health care and treatment of children and the study of childhood diseases is known as a ______________________________

46. A registered nurse with advanced study and clinical practice in pediatric nursing is known as a ______________________________

47. A routine health visit in which health professionals assess the current health status of the child, the progression of growth and development, and the need for immunizations is known as a ______________________________

48. The medical term for the top of the head is ______________________________

49. Telescoping of a portion of proximal intestine into distal intestine usually in the ileocecal region causing an obstruction, is known as ______________________________

50. A condition seen primarily in premature infants in which there is an abnormal opening between the pulmonary artery and the aorta caused by failure of the fetal ductus arteriosus to close after birth, is known as ______________________________

CHAPTER 19 ALTERNATE COMPLETION QUESTIONS

Emphasizing Word Elements and Abbreviations

(Can be substituted for Completion Questions 36-50)

COMPLETION

INSTRUCTIONS: Read each statement carefully and complete the statement with the most appropriate response. Enter your answer in the space provided.

36. The combining form **blast/o** means ______________________________

37. The combining form **cephal/o** means ______________________________

38. The combining form **crypt/o** means ______________________________

39. The prefix **epi-** means ______________________________

40. The combining form **hydr/o** means ______________________________

41. The combining form for **child** is ______________________________

42. The combining form for **navel** is ______________________________

43. The combining form for **heat, fire** is ______________________________

44. One combining form for **eardrum** is ______________________________

45. The prefix **hypo-** means ______________________________

46. The abbreviation for **sudden infant death syndrome** is ______________________________

47. The abbreviation for **Haemophilus influenzae type B** [vaccine] is ______________________________

48. The abbreviation for **measles-mumps-rubella** [vaccine] is ______________________________

49. The abbreviation for **phenylketonuria** is ______________________________

50. The abbreviation for **tuberculosis** is ______________________________

CHAPTER 20 RADIOLOGY AND DIAGNOSTIC IMAGING CHAPTER EXAM

MULTIPLE CHOICE

INSTRUCTIONS: The following questions or incomplete statements are followed by four answers or completions. Read each question carefully and select the most appropriate response.

1. An angiocardiography is also known as a(n)
   a. EKG
   b. cardiac catheterization
   c. cerebral angiography
   d. cineradiography
2. The injection of a radiopaque contrast medium into an arterial blood vessel to make visualization of the cerebral vascular system via x-ray possible, is known as a(n)
   a. cerebral angiography
   b. cerebral angioplasty
   c. CAT scan
   d. cholangiography
3. The x-ray visualization of the internal anatomy of the blood vessels of the kidney after injection of a contrast medium is known as a(n)
   a. cholangiography
   b. arthrography
   c. renal angiography
   d. nephropathy
4. The process of x-raying the inside of a joint, after a contrast medium has been injected into the joint is known as a(n)
   a. cholangiography
   b. arthrography
   c. renal angiography
   d. nephropathy
5. The infusion of a radiopaque contrast medium, into the rectum, that is held in the lower intestinal tract while x-rays are taken of the lower GI tract is known as a(n)
   a. barium swallow
   b. cholangiography
   c. barium enema
   d. nephrogram
6. A bronchial examination via x-ray following the coating of the bronchi with a radiopaque substance is known as a
   a. bronchography
   b. barium swallow
   c. cholangiography
   d. nephrography
7. Visualizing an outlining of the major bile ducts following an intravenous injection of a contrast medium is known as a(n)
   a. bronchography
   b. barium swallow
   c. cholangiography
   d. nephrography
8. The visualization of the gallbladder through x-ray following the oral ingestion of pills containing a radiopaque iodinated dye is known as a(n)
   a. cholecystography
   b. intravenous cholangiography
   c. barium swallow
   d. nephrogram
9. A painless, noninvasive diagnostic x-ray procedure using ionizing radiation that produces a detailed cross-sectional image of the body is known as a(n)
   a. ECRP
   b. echosomatography
   c. digital subtraction angiography
   d. computed axial tomography

10. X-ray visualization of the bladder and urethra during the voiding process, after the bladder has been filled with a contrast material is known as a(n)
    a. ECRP c. cystogram
    b. voiding cystourethrography d. KUB

11. X-ray images of blood vessels only, appearing without any background, due to the use of a computerized digital video process of subtraction is known as
    a. ECRP c. digital subtraction angiography
    b. echosomatography d. computed axial tomography

12. X-ray of the uterus and the fallopian tubes while filled with a contrast material is known as
    a. hysterosalpingography c. fallopianography
    b. hysterogram d. digital subtraction angiography

13. An x-ray assessment of the lymphatic system following an injection of a contrast medium into the lymph vessels in the hand or foot is known as a(n)
    a. MRI c. lymphangiography
    b. cholangiography d. myelography

14. The process of x-raying the soft tissue of the breast for the purpose of detecting benign and/or malignant growths before they can be felt is known as
    a. mammography c. myelography
    b. cystography d. MRI

15. The introduction of contrast medium into the lumbar subarachnoid space, through a lumbar puncture, in order to visualize the spinal cord and vertebral canal through x-ray examination is known as a(n)
    a. mammography c. myelography
    b. cystography d. MRI

16. An intravenous pyelogram, or pyelography, is also known as a(n)
    a. excretory urogram c. myelography
    b. cystography d. radioactive iodine uptake

17. Radiation therapy is the delivery of ionizing radiation to accomplish which of the following:
    1. destruction of tumor cells
    2. reduction of tumor size
    3. decrease in pain
    4. relief of obstruction
    5. to slow down or stop metastasis

    a. 1, 3, 5 only c. 2, 4, 5 only
    b. 1, 2, 3 only d. 1, 2, 3, 4 ,5

18. An examination that determines the position, size, shape, and physiological function of the thyroid gland through the use of radionuclear scanning is known as
    a. radioactive iodine uptake c. IVP
    b. MRI d. T6

19. Oral administration of a radiopaque contrast medium, barium sulfate, that flows through the GI system while x-ray films are obtained at timed intervals to observe the progression of the barium through the small intestine, is known as a(n)
    a. upper GI series c. ileogram
    b. small bowel follow-through d. barium sulfate series

20. The use of high-energy electromagnetic waves, passing through the body onto a photographic film, to produce a picture of the internal structures of the body for diagnosis and therapy is known as
    a. MRI c. cineradiography
    b. x-rays d. ultrasonography

MATCHING

INSTRUCTIONS: Match the term on the left with the correct definition on the right. Enter your selection in the space provided.

_____ 21. supine
_____ 22. anteroposterior
_____ 23. posteroanterior
_____ 24. eversion
_____ 25. inversion

a. a turning outward or inside out, such as a turning of the foot outward at the ankle
b. the direction from back to front
c. from the front to the back of the body
d. lying horizontally on the back
e. an abnormal condition in which an organ is turned inside out, or inward

_____ 26. lethal
_____ 27. nuclear medicine
_____ 28. palliative
_____ 29. radiographer
_____ 30. radiologist

a. to soothe or relieve
b. a medical discipline that uses radioactive isotopes in the diagnosis and treatment of disease
c. capable of causing death
d. a physician who specializes in radiology
e. an allied health professional trained to use x-ray machines and other imaging equipment to produce images of the internal structures of the body

_____ 31. radiology
_____ 32. radiolucent
_____ 33. radiopaque
_____ 34. tomography
_____ 35. teletherapy

a. radiation therapy administered by a machine that is positioned at some distance from the patient
b. not permitting the passage of x-rays or other radiant energy
c. pertaining to materials that allow x-rays to penetrate with a minimum of absorption
d. roentgenology
e. an x-ray technique that produces a film representing a detailed cross section of tissue structure at a predetermined depth

COMPLETION

INSTRUCTIONS: Read each statement carefully and complete the statement with the most appropriate response. Enter your answer in the space provided.

36. Placing a patient in a horizontal position, lying face downward, is known as what position?
____

37. Movement of a limb away from the body is known as _______________________

38. Movement of a limb toward the axis of the body is known as _______________________

39. Bending the elbow, to decreases the angle between the humerus and the ulna, is known as ______________________________

40. The treatment of neoplastic disease by using x-rays or gamma rays, to deter the proliferation of malignant cells by decreasing the rate of mitosis or impairing DNA synthesis, is known as ______________________________

41. Placing a patient in a lying down or leaning backward position is known as which position? ______________________________

42. A hand-held device that sends and receives a soundwave signal is known as a ______________

43. The drawing up or absorption of a substance is known as ______________________________

44. A radiographic process in which the aorta and its branches are injected with any of various contrast media for visualization is known as a(n) ______________________________

45. A method of radiographically visualizing the inside of a joint by injecting air or contrast medium is known as a(n) ______________________________

46. The placement of radioactive sources in contact with or implanted into the tissues to be treated is known as ______________________________

47. An x-ray examination of the bronchi after they have been coated with a radiopaque substance is known as a(n) ______________________________

48. The filming with a movie camera of the images that appear on a fluorescent screen is known as ______________________________

49. Exposure to any form of radiant energy like heat, light, or x-ray is known as ______________

50. The basic unit of absorbed dose of ionizing radiation is a ______________________________

CHAPTER 20 ALTERNATE COMPLETION QUESTIONS

Emphasizing Word Elements and Abbreviations

(Can be substituted for Completion Questions 36-50)

COMPLETION

INSTRUCTIONS: Read each statement carefully and complete the statement with the most appropriate response. Enter your answer in the space provided.

36. The combining form **angi/o** means ______________________________

37. The combining form **anter/o** means ______________________________

38. The combining form **arthr/o** means ______________________________

39. The combining form **arteri/o** means ______________________________

40. The combining form **chol/e** means ______________________________

41. The combining form **ech/o** means ______________________________

42. The prefix **cine-** means ______________________________

43. The combining form **fluor/o** means ______________________________

44. The combining form **poster/o** means ______________________________

45. The abbreviation for **computerized axial tomography** is ______________________________

46. The abbreviation for **chest x-ray** is ______________________________

47. The abbreviation for **fracture** is ______________________________

48. The abbreviation for **magnetic resonance imaging** is ______________________________

49. The abbreviation for **posteroanterior** is ______________________________

50. The abbreviation for **positron emission tomography** is ______________________________

CHAPTER 21 ONCOLOGY CHAPTER EXAM

MULTIPLE CHOICE

INSTRUCTIONS: The following questions or incomplete statements are followed by four answers or completions. Read each question carefully and select the most appropriate response.

1. Solid tumors, originating from epithelial tissue that make up the largest group of neoplasms are known as
   a. carcinomas
   b. lymphomas
   c. sarcomas
   d. adenomas
2. Tumors that originate from supportive and connective tissue such as bone, fat, muscle, and cartilage are known as
   a. carcinomas
   b. lymphomas
   c. sarcomas
   d. adenomas
3. A lifetime risk of developing cancer refers to
   a. the probability that an individual, over the course of his/her lifetime, will develop cancer or will die from cancer.
   b. measuring the strength of the relationship between risk factors and particular types of cancer, such as cigarette smoking.
   c. the projected age that an individual will develop cancer.
   d. the spread of cancer.
4. A relative risk of developing cancer refers to
   a. the probability that an individual, over the course of his/her lifetime, will develop cancer or will die from cancer.
   b. measuring the strength of the relationship between risk factors (such as cigarette smoking) and particular types of cancer.
   c. the projected age that an individual will develop cancer.
   d. the spread of cancer.
5. Which of the following are possible warning signs for the development of cancer?
   1. change in bowel of bladder habits
   2. sore that does not heal
   3. unusual bleeding or discharge
   4. obvious change in a wart or mole
   5. nagging cough or hoarseness

   a. 1, 2, 4, 5 only
   b. 2, 3, 4 only
   c. 1, 3, 4, 5 only
   d. 1, 2, 3, 4, 5
6. Bronchogenic carcinoma is also known as
   a. lung cancer
   b. basal cell carcinoma
   c. adenocarcinoma
   d. peau d'orange
7. The most common malignant tumor of the epithelial tissue that occurs most often on areas of the skin exposed to the sun is
   a. lung cancer
   b. basal cell carcinoma
   c. adenocarcinoma
   d. oral leukoplakia

8. A malignant tumor of the inner lining of the uterus is known as
   a. hysteroma
   b. endometrial carcinoma
   c. cervical carcinoma
   d. hydatidiform mole

9. A rare type of malignancy, associated with AIDS, that begins as soft purple-brown nodules or plaques on the feet, gradually spreading throughout the skin, is known as
   a. Kaposi's sarcoma
   b. Wilms' tumor
   c. malignant melanoma
   d. adenocarcinoma

10. A precancerous lesion occurring in the mouth, with gray white, leathery surfaced lesions, is known as
    a. malignant gingivitis
    b. polyps
    c. oral leukoplakia
    d. sarcoidosis

11. A darkly pigmented cancerous tumor, originating from melanocytes in pre-existing nevi, freckles, or skin with pigment, is called a
    a. malignant melonoma
    b. teratoma
    c. keratoma
    d. sarcoidosis

12. A malignant tumor of the kidney occurring predominately in childhood is known as
    a. Kaposi's sarcoma
    b. Wilms' tumor
    c. malignant melanoma
    d. astrocytoma

13. The use of cytotoxic drugs and chemicals to achieve a cure, decrease tumor size, provide relief of pain, or slow down metastasis, is known as
    a. radiation therapy
    b. adjuvant therapy
    c. chemotherapy
    d. fractionation

14. The use of ionizing radiation to interrupt cellular growth of a tumor is known as
    a. radiation therapy
    b. adjuvant therapy
    c. chemotherapy
    d. fractionation

15. An incision made into the body to remove a piece of a tumor for examination and diagnosing is called a(n)
    a. incisional biopsy
    b. excisional biopsy
    c. en bloc
    d. exenteration

16. The removal of the tumor and a portion of normal tissue for examination and diagnosis is called a(n)
    a. incisional biopsy
    b. excisional biopsy
    c. en bloc
    d. exenteration

17. A resection of a tumor and a large area of surrounding tissue that contains lymph nodes is called a(n)
    a. incisional biopsy
    b. excisional biopsy
    c. en bloc
    d. exenteration

18. The destruction of tissue by burning is known as
    a. cryosurgery
    b. electrocauterization
    c. dermabrasion
    d. exenteration

19. Treatment by freezing the malignant tissue that results in its destruction is known as
    a. cryosurgery
    b. electrocauterization
    c. dermabrasion
    d. exenteration

20. A wide resection that removes the organ or origin and surrounding tissue is called a(n)
    a. incisional biopsy
    b. excisional biopsy
    c. en bloc
    d. exenteration

MATCHING

INSTRUCTIONS: Match the term on the left with the correct definition on the right. Enter your selection in the space provided.

_____ 21. adjuvant
_____ 22. anaplasia
_____ 23. benign
_____ 24. carcinogen
_____ 25. carcinoma

a. a substance or agent that causes the development or increases the incidence of cancer
b. a malignant neoplasm
c. a substance, especially a drug, added to a prescription to assist in the action of the main ingredient
d. a change in the structure and orientation of cells, characterized by a loss of specialization and reversion to a more primitive form
e. noncancerous

_____ 26. carcinoma in situ
_____ 27. chemotherapy
_____ 28. invasive
_____ 29. encapsulated
_____ 30. infiltrative

a. enclosed in fibrous or membranous sheaths
b. characterized by a tendency to spread, infiltrate, and intrude
c. possessing the ability to invade or penetrate adjacent tissue
d. a premalignant neoplasm that has not invaded the basement membrane but shows cytologic characteristics of cancer
e. the use of chemical agents to selectively destroy cancer cells

_____ 31. fractionation
_____ 32. radiocurable
_____ 33. radioresponsive
_____ 34. radioresistant
_____ 35. radiotherapy

a. the treatment of disease by using x-rays or gamma rays
b. a tumor that resists the effects of radiation
c. a tumor that is capable of being destroyed by ionizing radiation
d. a tumor that reacts favorably to radiation
e. the division of the total dose of radiation into small doses administered at intervals, in an effort to minimize tissue damage

COMPLETION

INSTRUCTIONS: Read each statement carefully and complete the statement with the most appropriate response. Enter your answer in the space provided.

36. The process by which tumor cells spread to distant parts of the body is known as ____________________

37. A large nucleic acid molecule, found principally in the chromosomes of the nucleus of a cell, that is the carrier of genetic information is ____________________

38. High-energy x-rays with the ability to kill cells or retard their growth, are called ____________________

39. A type of cell division that results in the formation of two genetically identical daughter cells is known as ____________________

40. A growth composed of more than one kind of neoplastic tissue is called a ____________________

41. The medical term for a method of application, or a treatment method, is ______________________________

42. The medical term that refers to an illness or an abnormal condition or quality is ______________________________

43. The medical term that refers to a change or transformation is ______________________________

44. Any abnormal growth of new tissue, benign or malignant, is known as a(n) ______________________________

45. The medical term that refers to the formation of a tumor is ______________________________

46. The medical term that means pertaining to nipple-like projections is ______________________________

47. The medical term that means pertaining to a structure with a stalk is ______________________________

48. To exhibit again the symptoms of a disease from which a patient appears to have recovered is known as ______________________________

49. The partial or complete disappearance of the symptoms of a chronic or malignant disease is known as ______________________________

50. The medical term that means rough or warty is ______________________________

CHAPTER 21 ALTERNATE COMPLETION QUESTIONS

Emphasizing Word Elements and Abbreviations

(Can be substituted for Completion Questions 36-50)

COMPLETION

INSTRUCTIONS: Read each statement carefully and complete the statement with the most appropriate response. Enter your answer in the space provided.

36. The abbreviation for **metastasis** is ____________________

37. The abbreviation for **biopsy** is ____________________

38. The abbreviation for **prostate-specific antigen** is ____________________

39. The abbreviation for the **system for staging malignant neoplastic disease** is ____________________

40. The abbreviation for **ribonucleic acid** is ____________________

41. The combining form **carcin/o** means ____________________

42. The combining form **chem/o** means ____________________

43. The combining form **onc/o** means ____________________

44. The combining form **sarc/o** means ____________________

45. The combining form **scirrh/o** means ____________________

46. The prefix **ana-** means ____________________

47. The suffix **-blast** means ____________________

48. The prefix **meta-** means ____________________

49. The suffix **-oma** means ____________________

50. The combining form **papill/o** means ____________________

CHAPTER 22 PHARMACOLOGY CHAPTER EXAM

MULTIPLE CHOICE

INSTRUCTIONS: The following questions or incomplete statements are followed by four answers or completions. Read each question carefully and select the most appropriate response.

1. A life-threatening, hypersensitive reaction to a drug in which the patient experiences acute respiratory distress, hypotension, edema, tachycardia, cool, pale skin, cyanosis, and possibly convulsions shortly after administration of the medication is known as
   a. a localized reaction
   b. anaphylactic shock
   c. hives
   d. epilepsy
2. Any special symptom or circumstance that indicates that the use of a particular drug or procedure is dangerous, not advised, or has not been proven safe for administration, is known as
   a. a contraindication
   b. an idiosyncrasy
   c. a first-dose effect
   d. potentiation
3. When a drug level begins to accumulate in the body with repeated doses since the drug is not completely excreted from the body before another dose is administered, it is known as
   a. potentiation
   b. desired effect
   c. cumulation
   d. peak activity
4. The effect that was intended for a particular drug is known as the
   a. desired effect
   b. first-dose effect
   c. potentiation
   d. cumulation
5. An undesired effect of a medication that occurs within 30-90 minutes after administration of the first dose, is known as the
   a. potential effect
   b. cumulative effect
   c. first-dose effect
   d. peak activity
6. A response to a medication that is confined to a specific part of the body is known as the
   a. systemic effect
   b. local effect
   c. adverse effect
   d. cumulative effect
7. An unusual, potentially life-threatening, inappropriate response to a drug or to the usual effective dose of a drug, is known as a(n)
   a. idiosyncracy
   b. localized effect
   c. first-dose effect
   d. potentiated effect
8. The dose of a medication that will keep the concentration of the medication in the bloodstream at the desired level is known as the
   a. first dose
   b. controlled dose
   c. maintenance dose
   d. last dose
9. The effect that occurs when two drugs administered together produce a more powerful response than the sum of their individual effects, is known as
   a. potentiation
   b. toxic effect
   c. local effect
   d. idiosyncracy

10. An additional effect on the body by a drug that was not part of the goal for that medication, is known as a(n)
    a. cumulative effect
    b. side effect
    c. local reaction
    d. peak effect

11. The name under which the drug is sold by a specific manufacturer is called the
    a. chemical name
    b. brand name
    c. generic name
    d. controlled name

12. The description of the chemical structure of the drug is known as its
    a. chemical name
    b. brand name
    c. generic name
    d. controlled name

13. The name that is established when the drug is first manufactured, and is protected for use only by the original manufacturer for a period of 17 years, is known as the
    a. chemical name
    b. brand name
    c. generic name
    d. controlled name

14. The federal law that is concerned with the manufacture, distribution, and dispensing of drugs that have the potential of being abused and of causing physical or psychological dependence, is known as the
    a. Controlled Substance Act
    b. Food, Drug, and Cosmetic Act
    c. DEA
    d. FDA

15. A law that regulates the quality, purity, potency, effectiveness, safety, labeling, and packaging of food, drug, and cosmetic products, is the
    a. Controlled Substance Act
    b. Food, Drug, and Cosmetic Act
    c. DEA
    d. FDA

16. Drugs such as LSD, Heroin, and Marijuana, that are used for research only and are not considered to be legitimate for medical use in the United States, are classified as
    a. Schedule I drugs
    b. Schedule II drugs
    c. Schedule III drugs
    d. Schedule IV drugs

17. Drugs such as Robitussin A-C, Donnagel-PG, and Lomotil have a small potential for abuse or addiction, and are classified as
    a. Schedule I drugs
    b. Schedule II drugs
    c. Schedule IV drugs
    d. Schedule V drugs

18. The government agency responsible for administering and enforcing the Controlled Substances Act is the
    a. DEA
    b. FDA
    c. USP
    d. DFC

19. The government agency responsible for administering and enforcing the Food, Drug, and Cosmetic Act within the United States is the
    a. DEA
    b. FDA
    c. USP
    d. DFC

20. Rules that have been established to control the strength, quality, and purity of medications prepared by various manufacturers are known as
    a. standards
    b. pharmacopeias
    c. schedules
    d. drug facts and comparisons

MATCHING

INSTRUCTIONS: Match the term on the left with the correct definition on the right. Enter your selection in the space provided.

_____ 21. drug action	a. the change that takes place in the body as a result of a drug action
_____ 22. drug effect	b. the dose of a medication that achieves the desired effect
_____ 23. potency	c. the body's resistance to the effect of a drug
_____ 24. therapeutic dose	d. how a drug produces changes within the body
_____ 25. tolerance	e. strength

_____ 26. parenteral	a. medication that is placed in the mouth next to the cheek, where it is absorbed into the mucous membrane lining of the mouth
_____ 27. package insert	b. generic name
_____ 28. official name	c. an information leaflet placed inside the container or package of prescription drugs
_____ 29. trade name	d. any medication injected into the body using a needle and syringe
_____ 30. buccal medication	e. brand name

_____ 31. bacteriostatic	a. the study of how drugs interact in the human body
_____ 32. pharmacist	b. first dose
_____ 33. pharmacodynamics	c. stopping of controlling the growth of bacteria
_____ 34. pharmacology	d. one who is licensed to prepare and dispense drugs
_____ 35. initial dose	e. the field of medicine that specializes in the study of drugs, their sources, appearance, chemistry, actions, and uses

COMPLETION

INSTRUCTIONS: Read each statement carefully and complete the statement with the most appropriate response. Enter your answer in the space provided.

36. When repeated doses of a drug are given the drug starts to accumulate in the body tissues and toxic effects may occur; this is known as what type of effect? ______________________

37. A potentially life-threatening, unusual, inappropriate response to a drug or to the usual effective dose of a drug, is known a(n) ______________________

38. When two drugs administered together produce a more powerful response than the sum of their individual effects, it is called ______________________

39. The treatment of diseases using drugs that have a specific deadly effect on disease-causing microorganisms, as in the treatment of cancer, is known as ______________________

40. Any substance that, when taken into the body, may modify one or more of its functions, is known as a ______________________________

41. Another name for a druggist is a ______________________________

42. A reference book that lists all of the drugs commonly stocked in the hospital pharmacy is the ______________________________

43. Medication that is sprayed or breathed into the nose, throat, and lungs, is given by what route of administration? ______________________________

44. Medication that is inserted just beneath the epidermis using a syringe and needle is given by what route of administration? ______________________________

45. Medication that is injected directly into the vein, entering the bloodstream immediately is given by what route of administration? ______________________________

46. A reference book that provides the same information that is found in package inserts that accompanies each container of medication is the ______________________________

47. Medication that is applied directly to the skin or mucous membrane for a local effect to the area, is known as a ______________________________ medication.

48. A buccal medication is one that is placed in the mouth next to the cheek to be absorbed into the mucous membrane lining of the mouth is known as a ______________________________ medication.

49. The method of administering a drug to unbroken skin, in which the drug is absorbed continuously, producing a systemic effect, is known as ______________________________

50. A medication that is given to relieve pain is known as a(n) ______________________________

CHAPTER 22 ALTERNATE COMPLETION QUESTIONS

Emphasizing Word Elements and Abbreviations

(Can be substituted for Completion Questions 36-50)

COMPLETION

INSTRUCTIONS: Read each statement carefully and complete the statement with the most appropriate response. Enter your answer in the space provided.

36. The combining form **alges/o** means ______________________

37. The combining form **bucc/o** means ______________________

38. The combining form **chem/o** means ______________________

39. The combining form **esthesi/o** means ______________________

40. The combining form **gloss/o** means ______________________

41. The prefix **hypno-** means ______________________

42. The combining form **lingu/o** means ______________________

43. The combining form **pharmac/o** means ______________________

44. The combining form **toxic/o** means ______________________

45. The abbreviation for **before meals** is ______________________

46. The abbreviation for **as desired** is ______________________

47. The abbreviation for **twice a day** is ______________________

48. The abbreviation for **grain** is ______________________

49. The abbreviation for **drops** is ______________________

50. The abbreviation for **after meals** is ______________________

CHAPTER 23 MENTAL HEALTH CHAPTER EXAM

MULTIPLE CHOICE

INSTRUCTIONS: The following questions or incomplete statements are followed by four answers or completions. Read each question carefully and select the most appropriate response.

1. A state of frenzied excitement, that occurs rapidly and is characterized by difficulty maintaining and shifting attention, is known as
   a. delirium c. schizophrenia
   b. dementia d. depression

2. A psychological disorder characterized by episodes of mania, depression, alternating between the two, or a mixture of the two moods simultaneously, is known as
   a. paranoid schizophrenia c. bipolar disorder
   b. generalized anxiety disorder d. major depressive disorder

3. An anxiety disorder characterized by an obsessive, irrational, and intense fear of a specific object, of an activity, or of a physical situation, is known as
   a. psychogenic fugue c. schizophrenia
   b. phobic disorder d. hypochondriasis

4. One of the mood swings of the individual with bipolar disorder is characterized by extreme excitement, hyperactivity, agitation, overly talkative, flight of ideas, fleeting attention, and sometimes violent, destructive, and self-destructive behavior; this mood is known as
   a. mania c. excitability
   b. depression d. anxiety disorder

5. Another mood swing of the individual with bipolar disorder is characterized by exaggerated feelings of sadness, discouragement, and hopelessness that are inappropriate and out of proportion with reality; this mood is known as
   a. mania c. excitability
   b. depression d. anxiety disorder

6. A disorder characterized by chronic, unrealistic, and excessive anxiety and worry, with symptoms having been present for at least six months and having no relation to any specific causes, is known as
   a. major depressive disorder c. hypochondriasis
   b. phobic disorder d. generalized anxiety disorder

7. Repeated, persistent thoughts or impulses that are irrational and with which the mind is continually and involuntarily preoccupied, are known as
   a. obsessions c. manias
   b. compulsions d. depressions

8. A mental disorder in which the individual represses anxiety experienced by emotional conflicts by converting the anxious feelings into physical symptoms (such as paralysis or pain) that have no organic basis, but are perceived to be real by the individual, is known as
   a. subluxation c. conversion disorder
   b. Munchausen's syndrome d. cyclothymic disorder

9. An individual who has a chronic, abnormal concern about the health of his/her body, characterized by extreme anxiety, depression, and being preoccupied with a fear of having a serious illness or disease despite rational medical evidence that no disorder is present, would be classified as suffering from
   a. hypochondriasis
   b. Munchausen's syndrome
   c. cyclothymic disorder
   d. dissociative identity disorder

10. A somewhat rare form of child abuse in which a parent of a child falsifies an illness in a child by fabricating or creating the symptoms, and then seeks medical care for the child, is known as
    a. hypochondriasis (by proxy)
    b. Munchausen's syndrome (by proxy)
    c. cyclothymic disorder
    d. pedophilic syndrome

11. A sleep disorder that is characterized by a repeated, uncontrollable desire to sleep, often several times a day, is known as
    a. frotteurism
    b. dissociative amnesia
    c. narcolepsy
    d. dementia

12. A disorder in which there is the presence of two or more distinct personalities within one individual, is known as
    a. dissociative personality disorder
    b. paranoid schizophrenia
    c. frotteurism
    d. cyclothymic disorder

13. A disorder in which the individual is unable to recall important personal information, usually of a traumatic or stressful nature; the loss of memory is more than simple forgetting, is known as
    a. dissociative personality disorder
    b. dissociative amnesia
    c. dissociative fugue
    d. frotteurism

14. A sexual disorder involving the exposure of one's genitals to a stranger, is known as
    a. exhibitionism
    b. frotteurism
    c. fugue
    d. fetishism

15. A sexual disorder in which the individual is sexually aroused and engages in sexual activity with children (generally age 13 or younger), is called
    a. frotteurism
    b. fetishism
    c. pedophilia
    d. borderline personality

16. A disorder seen primarily in adolescent girls, characterized by an emotional disturbance concerning body image, prolonged refusal to eat followed by extreme weight loss, amenorrhea, and a lingering, abnormal fear of becoming obese, is known as
    a. anorexia nervosa
    b. fetishism
    c. bulimia nervosa
    d. hypochondriasis

17. An uncontrolled craving for food, often resulting in eating binges, followed by vomiting to eliminate the food from the stomach, is known as
    a. anorexia nervosa
    b. fetishism
    c. bulimia nervosa
    d. hypochondriasis

18. A personality disorder characterized by an extensive pattern of instability of interpersonal relationships, self-image, and marked impulsivity that begins by early adulthood and is present in a variety of contexts (such as gambling or binge eating), is known as
    a. frotteurism
    b. fetishism
    c. pedophilia
    d. borderline personality

19. A personality disorder characterized by an abnormal interest in oneself, especially in one's own body and sexual characteristics, is known as
    a. borderline personality disorder
    b. narcissistic personality disorder
    c. Munchausen's syndrome (by proxy)
    d. fetishism

20. A personality disorder characterized by a generalized distrust and suspiciousness of others, so much so that the individual blames them for his/her own mistakes and failures, is known as
    a. schizoid personality disorder
    b. paranoid personality disorder
    c. cyclothymic disorder
    d. borderline personality disorder

MATCHING

INSTRUCTIONS: Match the term on the left with the correct definition on the right. Enter your selection in the space provided.

_____ 21. compensation	a. the process of transferring a feeling or emotion from the original idea or object to a substitute idea or object
_____ 22. denial	b. the individual unconsciously identifies with another person or with some object
_____ 23. displacement	c. the act of transferring one's own unacceptable thoughts or feelings on to someone else
_____ 24. introjection	d. an effort to overcome, or make up for, real or imagined inadequacies
_____ 25. projection	e. a refusal to admit or acknowledge the reality of something, thus avoiding emotional conflict or anxiety

_____ 26. rationalization	a. rechanneling or redirecting one's unacceptable impulses and drives into constructive activities
_____ 27. regression	b. an involuntary blocking of unpleasant feelings and experiences from one's conscious mind
_____ 28. repression	c. attempting to make excuses or invent logical reasons to justify unacceptable feelings or behaviors
_____ 29. sublimation	d. a response to stress in which the individual reverts to an earlier level of development and the comfort measures associated with that level of functioning
_____ 30. suppression	e. the voluntary blocking of unpleasant feelings and experiences from one's mind

_____ 31. electroconvulsive therapy
_____ 32. family therapy
_____ 33. group therapy
_____ 34. hypnosis
_____ 35. draw-a-person test

a. a passive, trance-like state of existence that resembles normal sleep during which perception and memory are altered, resulting in increased responsiveness to suggestion
b. a personality test that is based on the interpretation of drawings of human figures of both sexes
c. the process of passing an electrical current through the brain to create a brief seizure in the brain, much like a spontaneous seizure from some forms of epilepsy
d. a form of psychotherapy that focuses the treatment on the process between family members that supports and sustains symptoms
e. the application of psychotherapeutic techniques within a small group of people who experience similar difficulties; also known as encounter groups

COMPLETION

INSTRUCTIONS: Read each statement carefully and complete the statement with the most appropriate response. Enter your answer in the space provided.

36. Loss of memory caused by severe emotional trauma, brain injury, substance abuse, or reaction to medications or toxins, is known as ______________________________

37. A state of mind in which the individual feels increased tension, apprehension, a painfully increased sense of helplessness, a feeling of uncertainty, fear, jitteriness, and worry, is known as ______________________________

38. Absence or suppression of observable emotion, feeling, concern, or passion, is known as ______________________________

39. A form of psychotherapy that seeks to modify observable, maladjusted patterns of behavior by substituting new responses to given stimuli, is known as ______________________________

40. An effort to overcome, or make up for, real or imagined inadequacies, is called ______________________________

41. Irresistible, repetitive, irrational impulses to perform an act; these behavior patterns intended to reduce anxiety, not provide pleasure or gratification, are known as ______________________________

42. An unconscious, intrapsychic reaction that offers protection to the self from a stressful situation is called a ______________________________

43. An acute and sometimes fatal psychotic reaction caused by cessation of excessive intake of alcoholic beverages over a long period of time, is known as ______________________________

44. A refusal to admit or acknowledge the reality of something, thus avoiding emotional conflict or anxiety, is known as ______________________________

45. A form of psychotherapy that focuses the treatment on the process between family members that supports and sustains symptoms, is called ______________________________

46. The spontaneous, consciously unrestricted association of ideas, feelings, or mental images, is known as ______________________________

47. A state of being characterized by impaired judgement, slurred speech, loss of coordination, irritability, and mood changes, possibly due to drugs or alcohol, is known as ______________________________

48. An ego defense mechanism whereby an individual unconsciously identifies with another person or with some object, assuming the supposed feelings and/or characteristics of the other personality or object, is known as ______________________________

49. A willful and deliberate faking of symptoms of a disease or injury to gain some consciously desired end, is known as ______________________________

50. The inability to speak because of a physical defect or emotional problem is known as ______________________________

CHAPTER 23 ALTERNATE COMPLETION QUESTIONS
Emphasizing Word Elements and Abbreviations

(Can be substituted for Completion Questions 36-50)

COMPLETION

INSTRUCTIONS: Read each statement carefully and complete the statement with the most appropriate response. Enter your answer in the space provided.

36. The combining form **iatr/o** means ______________________________

37. The suffix **-mania** means ______________________________

38. The combining form **ment/o** means ______________________________

39. The combining form **psych/o** means ______________________________

40. The combining form **schiz/o** means ______________________________

41. The suffix **-phobia** means ______________________________

42. The combining form **hypn/o** means ______________________________

43. The combining form **phil/o** means ______________________________

44. The suffix **-phoria** means ______________________________

45. The abbreviation for **attention deficit** is ______________________________

46. The abbreviation for *Diagnostic and Statistical Manual of Mental Disorders* is ____________

47. The abbreviation for **delirium tremens** is ______________________________

48. The abbreviation for **electroconvulsive therapy** is ______________________________

49. The abbreviation for **intelligence quotient** is ______________________________

50. The abbreviation for **Minnesota Multiphasic Personality Inventory** is ____________

ANSWER KEYS TO CHAPTER REVIEW SHEETS

CHAPTER 2: PREFIXES
ANSWERS TO CHAPTER REVIEW SHEET 1

WORD ELEMENT TO DEFINITION

WORD ELEMENT	DEFINITION
1. a-	*without, away from*
2. ab-	*from, away from*
3. ad-	*toward, increase*
4. alb-	*white*
5. ambi-	*both, both sides*
6. an-	*without, not*
7. ante-	*before, in front*
8. anti-	*against*
9. auto-	*self*
10. bi-	*two, double*
11. bio-	*life*
12. brady-	*slow*
13. circum-	*around*
14. con-	*together, with*
15. contra-	*against*
16. de-	*down, from*
17. dis-	*free of, to undo*
18. dys-	*bad, difficult*
19. ecto-	*outside*
20. endo-	*within*

CHAPTER 2: PREFIXES
ANSWERS TO CHAPTER REVIEW SHEET 2

DEFINITION TO WORD ELEMENT

DEFINITION	WORD ELEMENT
1. without, away from	*a- or an-*
2. from, away from	*ab-*
3. toward, increase	*ad-*
4. white	*alb-*
5. both, both sides	*ambi-*
6. without, not (different word from # 1)	*an- or a-*
7. before, in front	*ante-*
8. against	*anti- or contra-*
9. self	*auto*
10. two, double	*bi-*
11. life	*bio-*
12. slow	*brady-*
13. around	*circum-*
14. together, with	*con-*
15. against (different word from # 8)	*contra- or anti-*
16. down, from	*de-*
17. free of, to undo	*dis-*
18. bad, difficult	*dys-*
19. outside	*ecto-*
20. within	*endo- or intra-*

CHAPTER 2: PREFIXES
ANSWERS TO CHAPTER REVIEW SHEET 3

WORD ELEMENT TO DEFINITION

WORD ELEMENT	DEFINITION
1. epi-	*upon, over*
2. eu-	*good, normal*
3. ex-	*out, away from*
4. extra-	*outside of, beyond*
5. hemi-	*half*
6. homeo-	*likeness, same*
7. homo-	*same*
8. hydro-	*water*
9. hyper-	*excessive*
10. hypo-	*less than, under*
11. idio-	*individual*
12. in-	*in, within, not*
13. infra-	*beneath, under*
14. inter-	*between*
15. intra-	*within*
16. juxta-	*near, beside*
17. meta-	*change, after*
18. milli-	*one-thousandth*
19. mono-	*one, single*
20. multi-	*many*

CHAPTER 2: PREFIXES
ANSWERS TO CHAPTER REVIEW SHEET 4
DEFINITION TO WORD ELEMENT

DEFINITION	WORD ELEMENT
1. upon, over	*epi-*
2. good, normal	*eu-*
3. out, away from	*ex-*
4. outside of, beyond	*extra-*
5. half	*hemi- or semi-*
6. likeness, same	*homeo- or homo-*
7. same (different word from # 6)	*homo- or homeo-*
8. water	*hydro-*
9. excessive	*hyper-*
10. less than, under	*hypo-*
11. individual	*idio-*
12. in, within, not	*in-*
13. beneath, under	*infra-*
14. between	*inter-*
15. within	*intra- or endo-*
16. near, beside	*juxta-*
17. change, after	*meta-*
18. one-thousandth	*milli-*
19. one, single	*mono-*
20. many	*multi-*

CHAPTER 2: PREFIXES
ANSWERS TO CHAPTER REVIEW SHEET 5
WORD ELEMENT TO DEFINITION

WORD ELEMENT	DEFINITION
1. non-	*not*
2. pan-	*all*
3. para-	*near, beside*
4. per-	*through*
5. peri-	*around*
6. poly-	*many, much*
7. post-	*after, behind*
8. pre-	*before, in front*
9. primi-	*first*
10. pseudo-	*false*
11. retro-	*backward, behind*
12. semi-	*half*
13. sub-	*under, below*
14. supra-	*above, over*
15. sym-	*joined, together*
16. tachy-	*rapid*
17. trans-	*across, through*
18. tri-	*three*
19. uni-	*one*
20. xero-	*dry*

CHAPTER 2: PREFIXES
ANSWERS TO CHAPTER REVIEW SHEET 6
DEFINITION TO WORD ELEMENT

DEFINITION	WORD ELEMENT
1. not	*non-*
2. all	*pan-*
3. near, beside	*para-*
4. through	*per-*
5. around	*peri- or circum-*
6. many, much	*poly-*
7. after, behind	*post-*
8. before, in front	*pre-*
9. first	*primi-*
10. false	*pseudo-*
11. backward, behind	*retro-*
12. half	*semi- or hemi-*
13. under, below	*sub- or hypo-*
14. above, over	*supra-*
15. joined, together	*sym- or syn-*
16. rapid	*tachy-*
17. across, through	*trans-*
18. three	*tri-*
19. one	*uni- or mono-*
20. dry	*xero-*

CHAPTER 3: SUFFIXES
ANSWERS TO CHAPTER REVIEW SHEET 1
WORD ELEMENT TO DEFINITION

WORD ELEMENT	DEFINITION
1. -ac, -al	*pertaining to*
2. -ad	*toward*
3. -algesia	*sensitivity to pain*
4. -algia	*pain*
5. -ate	*something that*
6. -blast	*immature, embryonic*
7. -cele	*herniation*
8. -centesis	*surgical puncture*
9. -cide	*to kill*
10. -clasis	*crushing or breaking up*
11. -cyte	*cell*
12. -dynia	*pain*
13. -e, -a	*noun ending*
14. -ectasia	*stretching, dilatation*
15. -ectomy	*surgical removal*
16. -emia	*blood condition*
17. -er	*one who*
18. -esis	*condition of*
19. -genesis	*generating, formation*
20. -gram	*record or picture*

CHAPTER 3: SUFFIXES
CHAPTER REVIEW SHEET 2

DEFINITION TO WORD ELEMENT

DEFINITION	WORD ELEMENT
1. pertaining to	*-ac, -al*
2. toward	*-ad*
3. sensitivity to pain	*-algesia*
4. pain	*-algia, -dynia*
5. something that	*-ate*
6. immature; embryonic	*-blast*
7. herniation	*-cele*
8. surgical puncture	*-centesis*
9. to kill	*-cide*
10. crushing or breaking up	*-clasis*
11. cell	*-cyte*
12. pain (other than #4)	*-dynia, -algia*
13. noun ending	*-a, -e*
14. stretching, dilatation	*-ectasia*
15. surgical removal	*-ectomy*
16. blood condition	*-emia*
17. one who	*-er*
18. condition of	*-esis*
19. generating, formation	*-genesis*
20. record or picture	*-gram*

CHAPTER 3: SUFFIXES
CHAPTER REVIEW SHEET 3

WORD ELEMENT TO DEFINITION

WORD ELEMENT	DEFINITION
1. -graph	*instrument used to record*
2. -graphy	*process of recording*
3. -ia	*condition (other than -osis)*
4. -ion	*action*
5. -ist	*one who (a specialist in a field of study)*
6. -itis	*inflammation*
7. -lepsy	*seizure*
8. -lith	*stone*
9. -logy	*the study of*
10. -logist	*one who specializes in the study of*
11. -lysis	*destruction*
12. -mania	*madness*
13. -megaly	*enlargement*
14. -meter	*an instrument used to measure*
15. -metry	*the process of measuring*
16. -oid	*resembling*
17. -ole	*small or little*
18. -oma	*tumor*
19. -opia	*visual condition*
20. -osis	*condition (other than -ia)*

CHAPTER 3: SUFFIXES
ANSWERS TO CHAPTER REVIEW SHEET 4

DEFINITION TO WORD ELEMENT

DEFINITION	WORD ELEMENT
1. instrument used to record	*-graph*
2. process of recording	*-graphy*
3. condition	*-ia, -osis*
4. action	*-ion*
5. one who (a specialist in a field of study)	*-ist*
6. inflammation	*-itis*
7. seizure	*-lepsy*
8. stone	*-lith*
9. the study of	*-logy*
10. one who specializes in the study of	*-logist*
11. destruction	*-lysis*
12. madness	*-mania*
13. enlargement	*-megaly*
14. an instrument used to measure	*-meter*
15. the process of measuring	*-metry*
16. resembling	*-oid*
17. small or little	*-ole*
18. tumor	*-oma*
19. visual condition	*-opia*
20. condition (other than #3)	*-osis, -ia*

CHAPTER 3: SUFFIXES
ANSWERS TO CHAPTER REVIEW SHEET 5

WORD ELEMENT TO DEFINITION

WORD ELEMENT	DEFINITION
1. -pathy	*disease*
2. -penia	*decrease in, deficiency*
3. -pexy	*surgical fixation*
4. -philia	*attracted to*
5. -phobia	*abnormal fear*
6. -plasty	*surgical repair*
7. -plegia	*paralysis, stroke*
8. -pnea	*breathing*
9. -ptosis	*drooping, prolapse*
10. -rrhagia	*excessive flow, bursting forth*
11. -rrhaphy	*suturing*
12. -rrhea	*drainage, flow*
13. -rrhexis	*rupture*
14. -scope	*instrument used to view*
15. -stomy	*creation of a new opening*
16. -tomy	*incision into*
17. -tripsy	*crushing*
18. -uria	*a characteristic of urine*
19. -stasis	*stopping or controlling*
20. -scopy	*the process of viewing with an instrument*

CHAPTER 3: SUFFIXES
ANSWERS TO CHAPTER REVIEW SHEET 6
DEFINITION TO WORD ELEMENT

DEFINITION	WORD ELEMENT
1. disease	*-pathy*
2. decrease in, deficiency	*-penia*
3. surgical fixation	*-pexy*
4. attracted to	*-philia*
5. abnormal fear	*-phobia*
6. surgical repair	*-plasty*
7. paralysis, stroke	*-plegia*
8. breathing	*-pnea*
9. drooping, prolapse	*-ptosis*
10. excessive flow, bursting forth	*-rrhagia*
11. suturing	*-rrhaphy*
12. drainage, flow	*-rrhea*
13. rupture	*-rrhexis*
14. instrument used to view	*-scope*
15. creation of a new opening	*-stomy*
16. incision into	*-tomy*
17. crushing	*-tripsy*
18. a characteristic of urine	*-uria*
19. stopping or controlling	*-stasis*
20. the process of viewing with an instrument	*-scopy*

CHAPTER 4: WHOLE BODY TERMS
ANSWERS TO CHAPTER REVIEW SHEET 1
WORD ELEMENT TO DEFINITION

WORD ELEMENT	DEFINITION
1. abdomin/o	*abdomen*
2. anter/o	*front*
3. cervic/o	*neck*
4. coccyg/o	*coccyx*
5. crani/o	*skull, cranium*
6. cyt/o	*cell*
7. dors/o	*back*
8. umbilic/o	*navel*
9. thorac/o	*chest*
10. hist/o	*tissue*
11. ili/o	*ilium*
12. inguin/o	*groin*
13. sacr/o	*sacrum*
14. later/o	*side*
15. medi/o	*middle*
16. nucle/o	*nucleus*
17. pelv/i	*pelvis*
18. proxim/o	*near*
19. ventr/o	*belly, front side*
20. viscer/o	*internal organs*

CHAPTER 4: WHOLE BODY TERMS
ANSWERS TO CHAPTER REVIEW SHEET 2
DEFINITION TO WORD ELEMENT

DEFINITION	WORD ELEMENT
1. abdomen	*abdomin/o*
2. front	*anter/o*
3. neck	*cervic/o*
4. coccyx	*coccyg/o*
5. skull, cranium	*crani/o*
6. cell	*cyt/o*
7. back	*dors/o*
8. navel	*umbilic/o*
9. chest	*thorac/o*
10. tissue	*hist/o*
11. ilium	*ili/o*
12. groin	*inguin/o*
13. sacrum	*sacr/o*
14. side	*later/o*
15. middle	*medi/o*
16. nucleus	*nucle/o*
17. pelvis	*pelv/i*
18. near	*proxim/o*
19. belly, front side	*ventr/o*
20. internal organs	*viscer/o*

CHAPTER 5: INTEGUMENTARY SYSTEM
ANSWERS TO CHAPTER REVIEW SHEET 1
WORD ELEMENT TO DEFINITION

WORD ELEMENT	DEFINITION
1. adip/o	*pertaining to fat*
2. cutane/o	*skin*
3. derm/o	*skin*
4. dermat/o	*skin*
5. hidr/o	*sweat*
6. kerat/o	*horny*
7. lip/o	*fat*
8. erythr/o	*red*
9. leuk/o	*red*
10. melan/o	*black*
11. xanth/o	*yellow*
12. myc/o	*fungus*
13. onych/o	*nails*
14. pil/o	*hair*
15. scler/o	*hard*
16. squam/o	*scales*
17. trich/o	*hair*
18. xer/o	*dryness*
19. ichthy/o	*fish*
20. cauter/o	*burn*

CHAPTER 5: INTEGUMENTARY SYSTEM ANSWERS TO CHAPTER REVIEW SHEET 2

DEFINITION TO WORD ELEMENT

DEFINITION	WORD ELEMENT
1. pertaining to fat	*adip/o*
2. skin	*cutane/o, derm/o, dermat/o*
3. skin (other than #2)	*cutane/o, derm/o, dermat/o*
4. skin (other than #3)	*cutane/o, derm/o, dermat/o*
5. sweat	*hidr/o*
6. horny	*kerat/o*
7. fat	*lip/o*
8. red	*erythr/o*
9. white	*leuk/o*
10. black	*melan/o*
11. yellow	*xanth/o*
12. fungus	*myc/o*
13. nails	*onych/o*
14. hair	*pil/o, trich/o*
15. hard	*scler/o*
16. scales	*squam/o*
17. hair (other than #14)	*trich/o, pil/o*
18. dryness	*xer/o*
19. fish	*ichthy/o*
20. burn	*cauter/o*

CHAPTER 6: SKELETAL SYSTEM ANSWERS TO CHAPTER REVIEW SHEET 1

WORD ELEMENT TO DEFINITION

WORD ELEMENT	DEFINITION
1. acetabul/o	*acetabulum*
2. blast/o	*embryonic*
3. calc/i	*calcium*
4. calcane/o	*heel bone*
5. carp/o	*wrist*
6. -clast	*to break*
7. clavicul/o	*collar bone*
8. coccyg/o	*coccyx*
9. cost/o	*ribs*
10. crani/o	*skull*
11. femor/o	*femur*
12. fibul/o	*fibula*
13. gen/o	*produce*
14. humer/o	*humerus*
15. ili/o	*ilium*
16. ischi/o	*ischium*
17. kyph/o	*humpback*
18. lamin/o	*lamina*
19. lumb/o	*lower back*
20. -malacia	*softening*

CHAPTER 6: SKELETAL SYSTEM
CHAPTER REVIEW SHEET 2

DEFINITION TO WORD ELEMENT

DEFINITION	WORD ELEMENT
1. acetabulum	*acetabul/o*
2. embryonic	*blast/o*
3. calcium	*calc/i*
4. heel bone	*calcane/o*
5. wrist	*carp/o*
6. to break (suffix)	*-clast*
7. collar bone	*clavicul/o*
8. coccyx	*coccyg/o*
9. ribs	*cost/o*
10. skull	*crani/o*
11. femur	*femor/o*
12. fibula	*fibul/o*
13. produce	*gen/o*
14. humerus	*humer/o*
15. ilium	*ili/o*
16. ischium	*ischi/o*
17. humpback	*kyph/o*
18. lamina	*lamin/o*
19. lower back	*lumb/o*
20. softening (suffix)	*-malacia*

CHAPTER 6: SKELETAL SYSTEM
CHAPTER REVIEW SHEET 3

WORD ELEMENT TO DEFINITION

WORD ELEMENT	DEFINITION
1. mastoid/o	*mastoid process*
2. maxill/o	*upper jaw*
3. metacarp/o	*hand bones*
4. metatars/o	*foot bones*
5. myel/o	*bone marrow*
6. olecran/o	*elbow*
7. orth/o	*straight*
8. oste/o	*bone*
9. patell/o	*kneecap*
10. pelv/i	*pelvis*
11. phalang/o	*fingers, toes*
12. -physis	*growth, growing*
13. -porosis	*passage or pore*
14. pub/o	*pubis*
15. rach/i	*spinal column*
16. scoli/o	*crooked, bent*
17. spondyl/o	*vertebrae*
18. radi/o	*radius*
19. scapul/o	*shoulder blade*
20. tars/o	*ankle bones*

CHAPTER 6: SKELETAL SYSTEM
CHAPTER REVIEW SHEET 4

DEFINITION TO WORD ELEMENT

DEFINITION	WORD ELEMENT
1. mastoid process	*mastoid/o*
2. upper jaw	*maxill/o*
3. hand bones	*metacarp/o*
4. foot bones	*metatars/o*
5. bone marrow	*myel/o*
6. elbow	*olecran/o*
7. straight	*orth/o*
8. bone	*oste/o*
9. kneecap	*patell/o*
10. pelvis	*pelv/i*
11. fingers, toes	*phalang/o*
12. growth, growing (suffix)	*-physis*
13. passage or pore (suffix)	*-porosis*
14. pubis	*pub/o*
15. spinal column	*rach/i*
16. crooked, bent	*scoli/o*
17. vertebrae	*spondyl/o*
18. radius	*radi/o*
19. shoulder blade	*scapul/o*
20. ankle bones	*tars/o*

CHAPTER 7: MUSCLES AND JOINTS
CHAPTER REVIEW SHEET 1

WORD ELEMENT TO DEFINITION

WORD ELEMENT	DEFINITION
1. bucc/o	*cheek*
2. fasci/o	*band of fibrous tissue*
3. fibr/o	*fiber*
4. leiomy/o	*smooth muscle*
5. my/o	*muscle*
6. pector/o, thorac/o	*pertaining to the chest*
7. rhabdomy/o	*striated muscle*
8. tri-	*three*
9. troph/o	*development*
10. ankyl/o	*stiff*
11. arthr/o	*joint*
12. articul/o	*joint*
13. burs/o	*bursa*
14. ligament/o	*ligament*
15. oste/o	*bone*
16. ten/o	*tendon*
17. tendin/o	*tendon*
18. tend/o	*tendon*
19. electr/o	*electricity*
20. dors/o	*back*

CHAPTER 7: MUSCLES AND JOINTS
CHAPTER REVIEW SHEET 2

DEFINITION TO WORD ELEMENT

DEFINITION	WORD ELEMENT
1. cheek	*bucc/o*
2. band of fibrous tissue	*fasci/o*
3. fiber	*fibr/o*
4. smooth muscle	*leiomy/o*
5. muscle	*my/o*
6. pertaining to the chest	*pector/o, thorac/o*
7. striated muscle	*rhabdomy/o*
8. three (prefix)	*tri-*
9. development	*troph/o*
10. stiff	*ankyl/o*
11. joint	*arthr/o, articul/o*
12. joint (other than #11)	*arthr/o, articul/o*
13. bursa	*burs/o*
14. ligament	*ligament/o*
15. bone	*oste/o*
16. tendon	*ten/o, tendin/o, tend/o*
17. tendon (other than #16)	*ten/o, tendin/o, tend/o*
18. tendon (other than #17)	*ten/o, tendin/o, tend/o*
19. electricity	*electr/o*
20. back	*dors/o*

CHAPTER 8: NERVOUS SYSTEM
CHAPTER REVIEW SHEET 1

WORD ELEMENT TO DEFINITION

WORD ELEMENT	DEFINITION
1. cerebell/o	*cerebellum*
2. cerebr/o	*cerebrum*
3. encephal/o	*brain*
4. esthesi/o, -esthesia	*sensation or feeling*
5. gli/o	*pertaining to neuroglia cells*
6. kinesi/o, -kinesia	*movement*
7. myel/o	*spinal cord or bone marrow*
8. narc/o	*sleep*
9. neur/o	*nerve*
10. ton/o	*tension*
11. ventricul/o	*ventricle*
12. -sthenia	*strength*
13. thec/o	*sheath*
14. -phasia	*speech*
15. -lexia	*reading*
16. -lepsy	*seizure*
17. mening/o	*meninges*
18. narc/o	*sleep*
19. alges/o, -algesia	*sensitivity to pain*
20. -algia	*pain*

CHAPTER 8: NERVOUS SYSTEM
CHAPTER REVIEW SHEET 2

DEFINITION TO WORD ELEMENT

DEFINITION	WORD ELEMENT
1. cerebellum	*cerebell/o*
2. cerebrum	*cerebr/o*
3. brain	*encephal/o*
4. sensation or feeling	*esthesi/o, -esthesia*
5. pertaining to neuroglia cells	*gli/o*
6. movement	*kinesi/o, -kinesia*
7. spinal cord or bone marrow	*myel/o*
8. sleep	*narc/o*
9. nerve	*neur/o*
10. tension	*ton/o*
11. ventricle	*ventriucl/o*
12. strength (suffix)	*-sthenia*
13. sheath	*thec/o*
14. speech (suffix)	*-phasia*
15. reading (suffix)	*-lexia*
16. seizure (suffix)	*-lepsy*
17. meninges	*mening/o*
18. sleep	*narc/o*
19. sensitivity to pain	*alges/o, -algesia*
20. pain (suffix)	*-algia*

CHAPTER 9: BLOOD & LYMPHATIC SYSTEM
CHAPTER REVIEW SHEET 1

WORD ELEMENT TO DEFINITION

WORD ELEMENT	DEFINITION
1. agglutin/o	*to clump*
2. anis/o	*unequal*
3. bas/o	*base*
4. blast/o, -blast	*embryonic state of development*
5. chrom/o	*color*
6. coagul/o	*clotting*
7. cyt/o	*cell*
8. -emia	*blood condition*
9. eosin/o	*red, rosy*
10. erythr/o	*red*
11. -globin	*containing protein*
12. hem/o	*blood*
13. hemat/o	*blood*
14. kary/o	*nucleus*
15. morph/o	*form, shape*
16. phag/o, -phage	*to eat*
17. poikil/o	*varied, irregular*
18. sider/o	*iron*
19. spher/o	*round, sphere*
20. thromb/o	*clot*

CHAPTER 9: BLOOD & LYMPHATIC SYSTEM
CHAPTER REVIEW SHEET 2

DEFINITION TO WORD ELEMENT

DEFINITION	WORD ELEMENT
1. to clump	*agglutin/o*
2. unequal	*anis/o*
3. base	*bas/o*
4. embryonic state of development	*blast/o, -blast*
5. color	*chrom/o*
6. clotting	*coagul/o*
7. cell	*cyt/o*
8. blood condition (suffix)	*-emia*
9. red, rosy	*eosin/o*
10. red	*erythr/o*
11. containing protein (suffix)	*-globin*
12. blood	*hem/o, hemat/o*
13. blood (other than # 12)	*hem/o, hemat/o*
14. nucleus	*kary/o*
15. form, shape	*morph/o*
16. to eat	*phag/o, -phage*
17. varied, irregular	*poikil/o*
18. iron	*sider/o*
19. round, sphere	*spher/o*
20. clot	*thromb/o*

CHAPTER 10: CARDIOVASCULAR SYSTEM
CHAPTER REVIEW SHEET 1

WORD ELEMENT TO DEFINITION

WORD ELEMENT	DEFINITION
1. angi/o	*vessel*
2. aneurysm/o	*aneurysm*
3. arter/o	*artery*
4. arteri/o	*artery*
5. arteriol/o	*arteriole*
6. ather/o	*fatty*
7. cardi/o	*heart*
8. coron/o	*heart*
9. ech/o	*sound*
10. electr/o	*electrical*

CHAPTER 10: CARDIOVASCULAR SYSTEM
CHAPTER REVIEW SHEET 2

DEFINITION TO WORD ELEMENT

DEFINITION	WORD ELEMENT
1. vessel	*angi/o*
2. aneurysm	*aneurysm/o*
3. artery	*arter/o, arteri/o*
4. artery (other than #3)	*arter/o, arteri/o*
5. arteriole	*arteriol/o*
6. fatty	*ather/o*
7. heart	*cardi/o, coron/o*
8. heart (other than #7)	*cardi/o, coron/o*
9. sound	*ech/o*
10. electrical	*electr/o*

CHAPTER 11: RESPIRATORY SYSTEM
CHAPTER REVIEW SHEET 1

WORD ELEMENT TO DEFINITION

WORD ELEMENT	DEFINITION
1. alveol/o	*alveolus*
2. bronch/o	*bronchus*
3. epiglott/o	*epiglottis*
4. laryng/o	*larynx*
5. nas/o, rhin/o	*nose*
6. orth/o	*straight*
7. pector/o	*chest*
8. pharyng/o	*pharynx*
9. phren/o	*diaphragm*
10. pleur/o	*pleura*
11. pne/o	*breathing*
12. pneum/o	*lung, air*
13. pneumon/o	*lung, air*
14. pulmon/o	*lungs*
15. rhin/o, nas/o	*nose*
16. sinus/o	*sinus*
17. thorac/o	*chest*
18. trache/o	*trachea*
19. scop/o	*to view*
20. bronchiol/o	*bronchiole*

CHAPTER 11: RESPIRATORY SYSTEM
CHAPTER REVIEW SHEET 2

DEFINITION TO WORD ELEMENT

DEFINITION	WORD ELEMENT
1. alveolus	*alveol/o*
2. bronchus	*bronch/o*
3. epiglottis	*epiglott/o*
4. larynx	*laryng/o*
5. nose	*nas/o, rhin/o*
6. straight	*orth/o*
7. chest	*pector/o, thorac/o*
8. pharynx	*pharyng/o*
9. diaphragm	*phren/o*
10. pleura	*pleur/o*
11. breathing	*pne/o*
12. lung, air	*pneum/o, pneumon/o*
13. lung, air (other than #12)	*pneum/o, pneumon/o*
14. lungs	*pulmon/o*
15. nose (other than #5)	*rhin/o, nas/o*
16. sinus	*sinus/o*
17. chest (other than #7)	*thorac/o, pector/o*
18. trachea	*trache/o*
19. to view	*scop/o*
20. bronchiole	*bronchiol/o*

CHAPTER 12: DIGESTIVE SYSTEM
CHAPTER REVIEW SHEET 1

WORD ELEMENT TO DEFINITION

WORD ELEMENT	DEFINITION
1. amyl/o	*starch*
2. appendic/o, append/o	*appendix*
3. bil/i	*bile*
4. bucc/o	*cheek*
5. cec/o	*cecum*
6. cheil/o	*lips*
7. chol/e	*bile*
8. col/o	*colon*
9. colon/o	*colon*
10. dent/o	*tooth*
11. cholecyst/o	*gallbladder*
12. duoden/o	*duodenum*
13. -ectasia	*stretching*
14. -emesis	*to vomit*
15. enter/o	*intestines*
16. esophag/o	*esophagus*
17. gastr/o	*stomach*
18. gingiv/o	*gums*
19. gloss/o	*tongue*
20. gluc/o, glyc/o	*sugar, sweetness*

CHAPTER 12: DIGESTIVE SYSTEM
CHAPTER REVIEW SHEET 2

DEFINITION TO WORD ELEMENT

DEFINITION	WORD ELEMENT
1. starch	*amyl/o*
2. appendix	*appendic/o, append/o*
3. bile	*bil/i, chol/e*
4. cheek	*bucc/o*
5. cecum	*cec/o*
6. lips	*cheil/o*
7. bile (other than #3)	*chol/e, bil/i*
8. colon	*col/o, colon/o*
9. colon (other than #8)	*col/o, colon/o*
10. tooth	*dent/o*
11. gallbladder	*cholecyst/o*
12. duodenum	*duoden/o*
13. stretching (suffix)	*-ectasia*
14. to vomit (suffix)	*-emesis*
15. intestines	*enter/o*
16. esophagus	*esophag/o*
17. stomach	*gastr/o*
18. gums	*gingiv/o*
19. tongue	*gloss/o*
20. sugar, sweetness	*gluc/o, glyc/o*

CHAPTER 12: DIGESTIVE SYSTEM
CHAPTER REVIEW SHEET 3

WORD ELEMENT TO DEFINITION

WORD ELEMENT	DEFINITION
1. hepat/o	*liver*
2. ile/o	*ileum*
3. jejun/o	*jejunum*
4. lapar/o	*abdominal wall*
5. lingu/o	*tongue*
6. lip/o	*fat*
7. lith/o	*stone, calculus*
8. -lysis	*destruction*
9. mandibul/o	*mandible*
10. odont/o, dent/o	*teeth*
11. or/o	*mouth*
12. rect/o	*rectum*
13. peritone/o	*peritoneum*
14. -pepsia	*state of digestion*
15. sial/o	*saliva, salivary gland*
16. sigmoid/o	*sigmoid colon*
17. steat/o	*fat*
18. stomat/o	*mouth*
19. -tresia	*perforation*
20. -tripsy	*to crush*

CHAPTER 12: DIGESTIVE SYSTEM
CHAPTER REVIEW SHEET 4

DEFINITION TO WORD ELEMENT

DEFINITION	WORD ELEMENT
1. liver	*hepat/o*
2. ileum	*ile/o*
3. jejunum	*jejun/o*
4. abdominal wall	*lapar/o*
5. tongue	*lingu/o*
6. fat	*lip/o, steat/o*
7. stone, calculus	*lith/o*
8. destruction (suffix)	*-lysis*
9. mandible	*mandibul/o*
10. teeth	*odont/o, dent/o*
11. mouth	*or/o, stomat/o*
12. rectum	*rect/o*
13. peritoneum	*peritone/o*
14. state of digestion (suffix)	*-pepsia*
15. saliva, salivary gland	*sial/o*
16. sigmoid colon	*sigmoid/o*
17. fat (other than #6)	*steat/o, lip/o*
18. mouth (other than #11)	*stomat/o, or/o*
19. perforation (suffix)	*-tresia*
20. to crush (suffix)	*-tripsy*

CHAPTER 13: ENDOCRINE SYSTEM
CHAPTER REVIEW SHEET 1

WORD ELEMENT TO DEFINITION

WORD ELEMENT	DEFINITION
1. acr/o	*extremities*
2. aden/o	*gland*
3. andr/o	*male*
4. calc/o	*calcium*
5. cortic/o	*cortex*
6. crin/o, -crine	*secrete*
7. dips/o, -dipsia	*thirst*
8. kal/i	*potassium*
9. lact/o	*milk*
10. myx/o	*relating to mucus*
11. natr/o	*sodium*
12. oxy-	*sharp, quick*
13. pancreat/o	*pancreas*
14. somat/o	*body*
15. thyr/o, thyroid/o	*thyroid gland*
16. thym/o	*thymus gland*
17. toxic/o	*poisons*
18. -tropin	*stimulating effect of a hormone*
19. -uria	*urine condition*
20. gonad/o	*sex glands*

CHAPTER 13: ENDOCRINE SYSTEM
CHAPTER REVIEW SHEET 2

DEFINITION TO WORD ELEMENT

DEFINITION	WORD ELEMENT
1. extremities	*acr/o*
2. gland	*aden/o*
3. male	*andr/o*
4. calcium	*calc/o*
5. cortex	*cortic/o*
6. secrete	*crin/o, -crine*
7. thirst	*dips/o, -dipsia*
8. potassium	*kal/i*
9. milk	*lact/o*
10. relating to mucus	*myx/o*
11. sodium	*natr/o*
12. sharp, quick (prefix)	*oxy-*
13. pancreas	*pancreat/o*
14. body	*somat/o*
15. thyroid gland	*thyr/o, thyroid/o*
16. thymus gland	*thym/o*
17. poisons	*toxic/o*
18. stimulating effect of a hormone (suffix)	*-tropin*
19. urine condition (suffix)	*-uria*
20. sex glands	*gonad/o*

CHAPTER 14: SPECIAL SENSES
CHAPTER REVIEW SHEET 1

WORD ELEMENT TO DEFINITION

WORD ELEMENT	DEFINITION
1. ambly/o	*dull*
2. aque/o	*watery*
3. blephar/o	*eyelid*
4. corne/o	*cornea*
5. cor/o	*pupil*
6. conjunctiv/o	*conjunctiva*
7. dacry/o	*tears*
8. es/o	*within*
9. ex/o	*outward*
10. glauc/o	*gray, silver*
11. ir/o	*iris*
12. irid/o	*iris*
13. kerat/o	*cornea*
14. lacrim/o	*tears*
15. mi/o	*smaller*
16. nas/o	*nose*
17. ocul/o	*eye*
18. ophthalm/o	*eye*
19. -opia	*vision*
20. -opsia	*vision*

CHAPTER 14: SPECIAL SENSES
CHAPTER REVIEW SHEET 2

DEFINITION TO WORD ELEMENT

DEFINITION	WORD ELEMENT
1. dull	*ambly/o*
2. watery	*aque/o*
3. eyelid	*blephar/o*
4. cornea	*corne/o, kerat/o*
5. pupil	*cor/o*
6. conjunctiva	*conjunctiv/o*
7. tears	*dacry/o, lacrim/o*
8. within	*es/o*
9. outward	*ex/o*
10. gray, silver	*glauc/o*
11. iris	*ir/o, irid/o*
12. iris (other than #11)	*ir/o, irid/o*
13. cornea (other than #4)	*kerat/o, corne/o*
14. tears (other than #7)	*lacrim/o, dacry/o*
15. smaller	*mi/o*
16. nose	*nas/o*
17. eye	*ocul/o, ophthalm/o*
18. eye (other than #17)	*ophthalm/o, ocul/o*
19. vision (suffix)	*-opia, -opsia*
20. vision (suffix other than #19)	*-opsia, -opia*

CHAPTER 14: SPECIAL SENSES
CHAPTER REVIEW SHEET 3

WORD ELEMENT TO DEFINITION

WORD ELEMENT	DEFINITION
1. phac/o, phak/o	*lens*
2. phot/o	*light*
3. pupill/o, cor/o	*pupil*
4. retin/o	*retina*
5. scler/o	*hard*
6. vitre/o	*glassy*
7. xer/o	*dry*
8. acous/o	*hearing*
9. audi/o	*hearing*
10. labyrinth/o	*inner ear*
11. myring/o	*eardrum*
12. tympan/o	*eardrum*
13. ot/o	*ear*
14. scot/o	*darkness*
15. palpebr/o, blephar/o	*eyelid*
16. -ptosis	*drooping*
17. opt/o, optic/o	*eye, vision*
18. extra-	*outside of*
19. epi-	*upon*
20. hemi-	*half*

CHAPTER 14: SPECIAL SENSES
CHAPTER REVIEW SHEET 4
DEFINITION TO WORD ELEMENT

DEFINITION	WORD ELEMENT
1. lens	*phac/o, phak/o*
2. light	*phot/o*
3. pupil	*pupill/o, cor/o*
4. retina	*retin/o*
5. hard	*scler/o*
6. glassy	*vitre/o*
7. dry	*xer/o*
8. hearing	*acous/o, audi/o*
9. hearing (other than #8)	*audi/o, acous/o*
10. inner ear	*labyrinth/o*
11. eardrum	*myring/o, tympan/o*
12. eardrum (other than #11)	*tympan/o, myring/o*
13. ear	*ot/o*
14. darkness	*scot/o*
15. eyelid	*palpebr/o, blephar/o*
16. drooping (suffix)	*-ptosis*
17. eye, vision	*opt/o, optic/o*
18. outside of (prefix)	*extra-*
19. upon (prefix)	*epi-*
20. half (prefix)	*hemi-*

CHAPTER 15: URINARY SYSTEM
CHAPTER REVIEW SHEET 1
WORD ELEMENT TO DEFINITION

WORD ELEMENT	DEFINITION
1. albumin/o	*albumin*
2. azot/o	*nitrogen*
3. bacteri/o	*bacteria*
4. cali/o, calic/o	*calyx, calyces*
5. cyst/o	*urinary bladder*
6. dips/o	*thirst*
7. glomerul/o	*glomerulus*
8. ket/o, keton/o	*ketone bodies*
9. meat/o	*meatus*
10. noct/i	*night*
11. nephr/o	*kidney*
12. ren/o	*kidney*
13. olig/o	*scanty*
14. pyel/o	*renal pelvis*
15. py/o	*pus*
16. ureter/o	*ureter*
17. urethr/o	*urethra*
18. ur/o	*urine*
19. urin/o	*urine*
20. vesic/o	*urinary bladder*

CHAPTER 15: URINARY SYSTEM
CHAPTER REVIEW SHEET 2

DEFINITION TO WORD ELEMENT

DEFINITION	WORD ELEMENT
1. albumin	*albumin/o*
2. nitrogen	*azot/o*
3. bacteria	*bacteri/o*
4. calyx, calyces	*cali/o, calic/o*
5. urinary bladder	*cyst/o, vesic/o*
6. thirst	*dips/o*
7. glomerulus	*glomerul/o*
8. ketone bodies	*ket/o, keton/o*
9. meatus	*meat/o*
10. night	*noct/i*
11. kidney	*nephr/o, ren/o*
12. kidney (other than # 11)	*nephr/o, ren/o*
13. scanty	*olig/o*
14. renal pelvis	*pyel/o*
15. pus	*py/o*
16. ureter	*ureter/o*
17. urethra	*urethr/o*
18. urine	*ur/o, urin/o*
19. urine (other than # 18)	*ur/o, urin/o*
20. urinary bladder (other than #5)	*cyst/o, vesic/o*

CHAPTER 16: MALE REPRODUCTIVE SYSTEM
CHAPTER REVIEW SHEET 1

WORD ELEMENT TO DEFINITION

WORD ELEMENT	DEFINITION
1. balan/o	*glans penis*
2. crypt/o	*hidden*
3. epididym/o	*epididymis*
4. hydr/o	*water*
5. orchi/o, orch/o, orchid/o	*testicle*
6. semin/i	*semen*
7. sperm/o, spermat/o	*sperm*
8. prostat/o	*prostate gland*
9. vas/o	*vessel*
10. zo/o	*animal (man)*

CHAPTER 16: MALE REPRODUCTIVE SYSTEM CHAPTER REVIEW SHEET 2

DEFINITION TO WORD ELEMENT

DEFINITION	WORD ELEMENT
1. glans penis	*balan/o*
2. hidden	*crypt/o*
3. epididymis	*epididym/o*
4. water	*hydr/o*
5. testicle	*orchi/o, orch/o, orchid/o*
6. semen	*semin/i*
7. sperm	*sperm/o, spermat/o*
8. prostate gland	*prostat/o*
9. vessel	*vas/o*
10. animal (man)	*zo/o*

CHAPTER 17: FEMALE REPRODUCTIVE SYSTEM CHAPTER REVIEW SHEET 1

WORD ELEMENT TO DEFINITION

WORD ELEMENT	DEFINITION
1. -arche	*beginning*
2. cervic/o	*cervix*
3. colp/o	*vagina*
4. gynec/o	*woman*
5. hyster/o	*uterus*
6. mamm/o	*breast*
7. men/o	*menstruation*
8. metr/o, metri/o,	*uterus*
9. mast/o	*breast*
10. o/o	*egg, ovum*
11. oophor/o	*ovary*
12. -rrhea	*discharge, flow*
13. salping/o	*fallopian tubes*
14. vagin/o	*vagina*
15. vulv/o	*vulva*
16. uter/o	*uterus*
17. ovari/o	*ovary*
18. ov/o	*egg, ovum*
19. ante-	*before*
20. dys-	*bad, painful*

CHAPTER 17: FEMALE REPRODUCTIVE SYSTEM
CHAPTER REVIEW SHEET 2

DEFINITION TO WORD ELEMENT

DEFINITION	WORD ELEMENT
1. beginning (suffix)	*-arche*
2. cervix	*cervic/o*
3. vagina	*colp/o, vagin/o*
4. woman	*gynec/o*
5. uterus	*hyster/o, metr/o, metri/o, uter/o*
6. breast	*mamm/o, mast/o*
7. menstruation	*men/o*
8. uterus (other than #5)	*hyster/o, metr/o, metri/o, uter/o*
9. breast (other than #6)	*mamm/o, mast/o*
10. egg, ovum	*o/o, ov/o*
11. ovary	*oophor/o, ovari/o*
12. discharge, flow (suffix)	*-rrhea*
13. fallopian tubes	*salping/o*
14. vagina (other than #3)	*colp/o, vagin/o*
15. vulva	*vulv/o*
16. uterus (other than #5 or #8)	*hyster/o, metr/o, metri/o, uter/o*
17. ovary(other than #11)	*oophor/o, ovari/o*
18. egg, ovum (other than #10)	*o/o, ov/o*
19. before (prefix)	*ante-*
20. bad, painful (prefix)	*dys-*

CHAPTER 18: OBSTETRICS
CHAPTER REVIEW SHEET 1

WORD ELEMENT TO DEFINITION

WORD ELEMENT	DEFINITION
1. amni/o	*amnion*
2. ante-	*before*
3. culd/o	*vagina*
4. -cyesis	*pregnancy*
5. episi/o	*vulva*
6. fet/o	*fetus*
7. -gravida	*pregnancy*
8. hyper-	*excessive, high*
9. lact/o	*milk*
10. multi-	*many*
11. nat/o	*birth*
12. nulli-	*none*
13. -para	*to give birth*
14. primi-	*first*
15. obstetr/o	*midwife*
16. perine/o	*perineum*
17. salping/o	*fallopian tube*
18. -tocia	*labor*
19. vagin/o	*vagina*
20. pelv/i	*pelvis*

CHAPTER 18: OBSTETRICS
CHAPTER REVIEW SHEET 2

DEFINITION TO WORD ELEMENT

DEFINITION	WORD ELEMENT
1. amnion	*amni/o*
2. before (prefix)	*ante-*
3. vagina	*culd/o, vagin/o*
4. pregnancy (suffix)	*-cyesis, -gravida*
5. vulva	*episi/o*
6. fetus	*fet/o*
7. pregnancy (suffix)	*-cyesis, -gravida*
8. excessive, high (prefix)	*hyper-*
9. milk	*lact/o*
10. many (prefix)	*multi-*
11. birth	*nat/o*
12. none (prefix)	*nulli-*
13. to give birth (suffix)	*-para*
14. first (prefix)	*primi-*
15. midwife	*obstetr/o*
16. perineum	*perine/o*
17. fallopian tube	*salping/o*
18. labor (suffix)	*-tocia*
19. vagina (other than #3)	*culd/o, vagin/o*
20. pelvis	*pelv/i*

CHAPTER 19: CHILD HEALTH
CHAPTER REVIEW SHEET 1

WORD ELEMENT TO DEFINITION

WORD ELEMENT	DEFINITION
1. cephal/o	*head*
2. crypt/o	*hidden*
3. hydr/o	*water*
4. hypo-	*under*
5. micr/o	*small*
6. ne/o	*new*
7. omphal/o	*navel*
8. pedi/a	*child*
9. pyr/o	*heat, fire*
10. tetr/a	*four*

CHAPTER 19: CHILD HEALTH
CHAPTER REVIEW SHEET 2

DEFINITION TO WORD ELEMENT

DEFINITION	WORD ELEMENT
1. head	*cephal/o*
2. hidden	*crypt/o*
3. water	*hydr/o*
4. under (prefix)	*hypo-*
5. small	*micr/o*
6. new	*ne/o*
7. navel	*omphal/o*
8. child	*pedi/a*
9. heat, fire	*pyr/o*
10. four	*tetr/a*

CHAPTER 20: RADIOLOGY & DIAGNOSTIC IMAGING
CHAPTER REVIEW SHEET 1

WORD ELEMENT TO DEFINITION

WORD ELEMENT	DEFINITION
1. angi/o	*vessel*
2. anter/o	*front*
3. arthr/o	*joint*
4. arteri/o	*artery*
5. cardi/o	*heart*
6. chol/e	*gall, bile*
7. cine-	*pertaining to movement*
8. ech/o	*sound*
9. fluor/o	*luminous*
10. lymph/o	*lymph*
11. myel/o	*bone marrow, spinal cord*
12. poster/o	*back*
13. pyel/o	*renal pelvis*
14. radi/o	*radiation, x-ray*
15. son/o	*sound*
16. tel/e	*distance*
17. tom/o	*to cut, section*
18. ultra-	*beyond*
19. ven/o	*vein*
20. xer/o	*dry*

CHAPTER 20: RADIOLOGY & DIAGNOSTIC IMAGING
CHAPTER REVIEW SHEET 2

DEFINITION TO WORD ELEMENT

DEFINITION	WORD ELEMENT
1. vessel	*angi/o*
2. front	*anter/o*
3. joint	*arthr/o*
4. artery	*arteri/o*
5. heart	*cardi/o*
6. gall, bile	*chol/e*
7. pertaining to movement (prefix)	*cine-*
8. sound	*ech/o*
9. luminous	*fluor/o*
10. lymph	*lymph/o*
11. bone marrow, spinal cord	*myel/o*
12. back	*poster/o*
13. renal pelvis	*pyel/o*
14. radiation, x-ray	*radi/o*
15. sound (other than # 8)	*son/o*
16. distance	*tel/e*
17. to cut; section	*tom/o*
18. beyond (prefix)	*ultra-*
19. vein	*ven/o*
20. dry	*xer/o*

CHAPTER 21: ONCOLOGY
CHAPTER REVIEW SHEET 1

WORD ELEMENT TO DEFINITION

WORD ELEMENT	DEFINITION
1. ana-	*not, without*
2. -blast	*embryonic state of development*
3. carcin/o	*cancer*
4. chem/o	*pertaining to a chemical*
5. meta-	*change*
6. -oma	*tumor*
7. onc/o	*tumor*
8. sarc/o	*of or related to flesh*
9. scirrh/o	*hard*
10. -plasia	*formation or development*

CHAPTER 21: ONCOLOGY
CHAPTER REVIEW SHEET 2

DEFINITION TO WORD ELEMENT

DEFINITION	WORD ELEMENT
1. not, without (prefix)	*ana-*
2. embryonic state of development (suffix)	*-blast*
3. cancer	*carcin/o*
4. pertaining to a chemical	*chem/o*
5. change (prefix)	*meta-*
6. tumor (suffix)	*-oma*
7. tumor (other than # 6)	*onc/o*
8. of or related to flesh	*sarc/o*
9. hard	*scirrh/o*
10. formation or development (suffix)	*-plasia*

CHAPTER 22: PHARMACOLOGY
CHAPTER REVIEW SHEET 1

MENT TO DEFINITION

WORD ELEMENT	DEFINITION
1. alges/o	*pain*
2. anti-	*against*
3. arrhythm/o	*rhythm*
4. bi/o	*life*
5. bucc/o	*cheek*
6. chem/o	*drug*
7. coagul/o	*clotting*
8. ven/o	*vein*
9. esthesi/o	*feeling*
10. fung/o	*fungus*
11. gloss/o	*tongue*
12. hyper-	*excessive, high*
13. hypno-	*sleep*
14. vagin/o	*vagina*
15. rect/o	*rectum*
16. -ist	*specialist*
17. lingu/o	*tongue*
18. -logy	*the study of*
19. toxic/o	*poison*
20. or/o	*mouth*

CHAPTER 22: PHARMACOLOGY
CHAPTER REVIEW SHEET 2

DEFINITION TO WORD ELEMENT

DEFINITION	WORD ELEMENT
1. pain	*alges/o*
2. against (prefix)	*anti-*
3. rhythm	*arrhythm/o*
4. life	*bi/o*
5. cheek	*bucc/o*
6. drug	*chem/o*
7. clotting	*coagul/o*
8. vein	*ven/o*
9. feeling	*esthesi/o*
10. fungus	*fung/o*
11. tongue	*gloss/o, lingu/o*
12. excessive, high (prefix)	*hyper-*
13. sleep (prefix)	*hypno-*
14. vagina	*vagin/o*
15. rectum	*rect/o*
16. specialist (suffix)	*-ist*
17. tongue (other than # 11)	*lingu/o, gloss/o*
18. the study of (suffix)	*-logy*
19. poison	*toxic/o*
20. mouth	*or/o*

CHAPTER 23: MENTAL HEALTH
CHAPTER REVIEW SHEET 1

WORD ELEMENT TO DEFINITION

WORD ELEMENT	DEFINITION
1. cata-	*down, under, against, lower*
2. hypn/o	*sleep*
3. iatr/o	*pertaining to a physician or treatment*
4. -mania	*madness*
5. ment/o	*mind*
6. phil/o	*having a love for or a strong attraction to*
7. -phobia	*abnormal fear*
8. -phoria	*emotional state*
9. psych/o	*mind*
10. schiz/o	*split, divided*

CHAPTER 23: MENTAL HEALTH
CHAPTER REVIEW SHEET 2

DEFINITION TO WORD ELEMENT

DEFINITION	WORD ELEMENT
1. down, under, against, lower (prefix)	*cata-*
2. sleep	*hypn/o*
3. pertaining to a physician or treatment	*iatr/o*
4. madness (suffix)	*-mania*
5. mind	*ment/o, psych/o*
6. having a love for or a strong attraction to	*phil/o*
7. abnormal fear (suffix)	*-phobia*
8. emotional state (suffix)	*-phoria*
9. mind (other than #5)	*ment/o, psych/o*
10. split, divided	*schiz/o*

ANSWER KEYS TO CHAPTER EXAMS

CHAPTER 1: WORD BUILDING RULES

NO EXAM FOR THIS CHAPTER

CHAPTER 2: PREFIXES

1. a
2. a
3. b
4. c
5. d
6. b
7. c
8. a
9. b
10. d
11. b
12. a
13. c
14. a
15. b
16. c
17. d
18. b
19. a
20. d
21. b
22. d
23. c
24. e
25. a
26. b
27. e
28. d
29. c
30. a
31. b
32. d
33. a
34. c
35. e
36. many, much
37. after, behind
38. before, in front
39. first
40. false
41. backward, behind
42. under, below
43. above, over
44. sym- , syn-
45. tachy-
46. trans-
47. tri-
48. uni-, mono-
49. xero-
50. peri-, circum-

CHAPTER 3: SUFFIXES

1. b
2. a
3. b
4. c
5. d
6. b
7. b
8. a
9. c
10. a
11. d
12. b
13. c
14. b
15. a
16. d
17. a
18. c
19. a
20. d
21. b
22. c
23. e
24. d
25. a
26. c
27. d
28. a
29. e
30. b
31. b
32. d
33. c
34. e
35. a
36. disease
37. decrease in; deficiency
38. surgical fixation
39. attracted to
40. abnormal fear
41. surgical repair
42. paralysis; stroke
43. -pnea
44. -ptosis
45. -rrhaphy
46. -rrhea
47. -rrhexis
48. -tomy
49. -stomy
50. -tripsy

CHAPTER 4: WHOLE BODY TERMS

1. b
2. d
3. a
4. b
5. c
6. b
7. d
8. a
9. a
10. b
11. c
12. d
13. a
14. b
15. c
16. a
17. b
18. d
19. a
20. c
21. b
22. c
23. a
24. e
25. d
26. d
27. e
28. c
29. b
30. a
31. c
32. d
33. e
34. a
35. b
36. front
37. cell
38. tissue
39. groin
40. side
41. back
42. near
43. belly; front side
44. ana-
45. cervic/o
46. hypo-
47. inter-
48. medi/o
49. umbilic/o
50. epi-

CHAPTER 5: INTEGUMENTARY SYSTEM

1. a
2 b
3. d
4. c
5. d
6. a
7. b
8. c
9. a
10. a
11. c
12. d
13. b
14. a
15. b
16. a
17. b
18. d
19. a
20. d
21. b
22. e
23. d
24. c
25. a
26. b
27. a
28. d
29. e
30. c
31. a
32. d
33. b
34. e
35. c
36. ulcer
37. sweat, perspiration
38. sweat gland
39. subcutaneous tissue
40. stretch marks
41. sebum
42. pruritus
43. pediculosis
44. lanula
45. laceration
46. hair follicle
47. epidermis
48. dermatologist
49. corium
50. cellulitis

ANSWERS TO ALTERNATE COMPLETION QUESTIONS

36. skin
37. skin
38. horny
39. fat
40. black
41. fungus
42. nails
43. ichthy/o
44. xanth/o
45. leuk/o
46. Bx
47. ID
48. I&D
49. PPD
50. ung.

CHAPTER 6: SKELETAL SYSTEM

1. a
2. b
3. a
4. a
5. c
6. d
7. a
8. a
9. b
10. b
11. a
12. c
13. d
14. a
15. c
16. b
17. a
18. c
19. b
20. d
21. c
22. d
23. e
24. b
25. a
26. d
27. e
28. a
29. c
30. b
31. c
32. d
33. a
34. e
35. b
36. suture
37. epiphysis
38. osteomyelitis
39. temporal bones
40. lacrimal bones
41. false ribs
42. intercostal spaces
43. ossification
44. osteocytes
45. osteomalacia
46. impacted
47. Colle's
48. stress
49. pathological
50. open reduction

ANSWERS TO ALTERNATE COMPLETION QUESTIONS

36. bone
37. vertebra
38. humpback
39. curve, swayback
40. crooked, bent
41. ribs
42. osteomyelitis
43. acromion
44. broken bone, no open wound in the skin
45. bone is broken on one side, bent on the other
46. DEXA
47. Fx
48. L2
49. TKR
50. TMJ

CHAPTER 7: MUSCLES AND JOINTS

1. a
2 d
3. b
4. b
5. d
6. a
7. c
8. a
9. a
10. b
11. a
12. a
13. b
14. b
15. a
16. b
17. c
18. a
19. b
20. a
21. c
22. e
23. d
24. b
25. a
26. b
27. d
28. e
29. a
30. c
31. c
32. d
33. e
34. b
35. a
36. arthralgia
37. contracture
38. torso
39. atrophy
40. fascia
41. ball-and-socket
42. synovial fluid
43. sciatica
44. sticky
45. photosensitivity
46. subluxation
47. involuntary muscles
48. pelvic girdle weakness
49. bunionectomy
50. suture

ANSWERS TO ALTERNATE COMPLETION QUESTIONS

36. cheek
37. band of fibrous tissue
38. fiber
39. smooth muscle
40. muscle
41. pertaining to the chest
42. development
43. three
44. ankyl/o
45. arthr/o
46. LLE
47. MCP
48. RA
49. SED RATE
50. SLE

CHAPTER 8: NERVOUS SYSTEM

1. b
2 a
3. c
4. b
5. d
6. a
7. b
8. c
9. d
10. a
11. c
12. a
13. b
14. c
15. c
16. b
17. d
18. a
19. b
20. c
21. d
22. e
23. c
24. a
25. b
26. b
27. e
28. d
29. a
30. c
31. c
32. e
33. b
34. d
35. a
36. afferent
37. brain stem
38. burr hole
39. cerebellum
40. contusion
41. cerebrospinal fluid
42. coma
43. craniotomy
44. deficit
45. dysphasia
46. hemiplegia
47. hyperesthesia
48. medulla oblongata
49. meninges
50. narcolepsy

ANSWERS TO ALTERNATE COMPLETION QUESTIONS

36. sensitivity to pain
37. pain
38. slow
39. brain
40. sensation or feeling
41. pertaining to neuroglial cells
42. movement
43. seizure
44. -lexia
45. myel/o
46. CNS
47. CVA
48. EEG
49. ICP
50. PET

CHAPTER 9: BLOOD & LYMPHATIC SYSTEM

1. b
2 b
3. d
4. b
5. a
6. c
7. b
8. d
9. a
10. b
11. a
12. b
13. c
14. b
15. d
16. a
17. b
18. b
19. a
20. c
21. c
22. e
23. d
24. a
25. b
26. d
27. e
28. b
29. a
30. c
31. d
32. b
33. e
34. a
35. c
36. allergen
37. coagulation
38. edema
39. pancytopenia
40. septicemia
41. splenomegaly
42. thrombocyte
43. thrombus
44. embolus
45. antigen
46. acquired immunity
47. natural immunity
48. pathogens
49. susceptible
50. local

ANSWERS TO ALTERNATE COMPLETION QUESTIONS

36. to clump
37. color
38. cell
39. blood condition
40. red, rosy
41. stopping or controlling
42. hem/o, hemat/o
43. form, shape
44. -penia
45. -phage
46. CBC
47. Hb, Hbg, Hgb
48. Hct
49. CDC
50. HIV

CHAPTER 10: CARDIOVASCULAR SYSTEM

1. b
2. a
3. c
4. b
5. d
6. a
7. c
8. a
9. b
10. d
11. c
12. a
13. d
14. b
15. a
16. b
17. a
18. a
19. c
20. a
21. c
22. e
23. d
24. a
25. b
26. c
27. e
28. a
29. d
30. b
31. b
32. c
33. d
34. a
35. e
36. aneurysm
37. cusp
38. diastole
39. abnormal rhythm
40. endocarditis
41. hypotension
42. mediastinum
43. pulmonary arteries
44. pacemaker
45. systemic
46. pulmonary
47. systole
48. vasoconstriction
49. vegetation
50. hypertension

ANSWERS TO ALTERNATE COMPLETION QUESTIONS

36. vessel
37. fatty
38. heart
39. heart
40. sound
41. electrical
42. within
43. to record
44. megal/o
45. my/o
46. BBB
47. ASHD
48. HCVD
49. CHF
50. MI

CHAPTER 11: RESPIRATORY SYSTEM

1. a
2. c
3. a
4. c
5. a
6. b
7. c
8. d
9. b
10. c
11. d
12. b
13. c
14. b
15. c
16. a
17. a
18. b
19. d
20. b
21. e
22. c
23. d
24. b
25. a
26. e
27. d
28. a
29. b
30. c
31. e
32. c
33. d
34. a
35. b
36. apex
37. base
38. voice box
39. windpipe
40. nasopharynx
41. pleura
42. chest
43. throat
44. nares
45. epiglottis
46. diaphragm
47. bronchi
48. alveoli
49. paranasal sinuses
50. visceral

ANSWERS TO ALTERNATE COMPLETION QUESTIONS

36. alveolus
37. bronchus
38. larynx
39. chest
40. diaphragm
41. lungs
42. breathing
43. lung, air
44. rhin/o, nas/o
45. thorac/o
46. shortness of breath
47. sudden infant death syndrome
48. left lower lobe (of the lung)
49. intermittent positive pressure breathing
50. chronic obstructive pulmonary disease

CHAPTER 12: DIGESTIVE SYSTEM

1. b
2. a
3. b
4. c
5. a
6. b
7. c
8. a
9. b
10. a
11. d
12. c
13. a
14. d
15. a
16. c
17. d
18. a
19. b
20. c
21. c
22. d
23. e
24. b
25. a
26. d
27. e
28. a
29. c
30. b
31. c
32. d
33. a
34. e
35. b
36. amylase
37. bile
38. gastroenterologist
39. chyme
40. crown
41. deciduous teeth
42. defecation
43. dietitian
44. digestion
45. enamel
46. endocrine gland
47. exocrine gland
48. gavage
49. gingiva
50. glucagon

ANSWERS TO ALTERNATE COMPLETION QUESTIONS

36. starch
37. enzyme
38. bile
39. lips
40. stretching, dilatation
41. to vomit
42. intestines
43. mouth
44. gingiv/o
45. gloss/o, lingu/o
46. hepat/o
47. gastr/o
48. -tresia
49. sigmoid/o
50. sial/o

CHAPTER 13: ENDOCRINE SYSTEM

1. a
2. c
3. b
4. a
5. b
6. a
7. a
8. b
9. b
10. a
11. b
12. c
13. b
14. a
15. c
16. a
17. c
18. b
19. a
20. c
21. d
22. e
23. b
24. c
25. a
26. a
27. d
28. e
29. b
30. c
31. b
32. c
33. d
34. e
35. a
36. medulla
37. metabolism
38. polydipsia
39. oxytocin
40. growth hormone
41. syndrome
42. tetany
43. serum glucose tests
44. thyroid scan
45. hyperinsulinism
46. endocrinology
47. hypocalcemia
48. glucagon
49. glycogenolysis
50. androgens

ANSWERS TO ALTERNATE COMPLETION QUESTIONS

36. extremities
37. gland
38. calcium
39. cortex
40. secrete
41. thirst
42. potassium
43. sodium
44. glyc/o, gluc/o
45. toxic/o
46. FBS
47. ACTH
48. IDDM
49. K
50. Na

CHAPTER 14: SPECIAL SENSES

1. b
2. a
3. c
4. d
5. a
6. a
7. b
8. a
9. a
10. b
11. c
12. b
13. d
14. d
15. c
16. d
17. a
18. a
19. a
20. c

21. d
22. c
23. e
24. a
25. b
26. e
27. c
28. d
29. b
30. a
31. d
32. e
33. a
34. b
35. c
36. retinopathy
37. acoustic
38. audiometry
39. mastoiditis
40. otitis media
41. presbycusis
42. myringoplasty
43. vertigo
44. labrinthitis
45. swimmer's ear
46. otosclerosis
47. otoscopy
48. otoplasty
49. ophthalmologist
50. ophthalmoscope

ANSWERS TO ALTERNATE COMPLETION QUESTIONS

36. both
37. dull
38. pupil
39. tears
40. -ptosis
41. vitre/o
42. tympan/o, myring/o
43. audi/o, acous/o
44. AU
45. dB
46. EENT
47. BOM
48. EOM
49. IOP
50. OD

CHAPTER 15: URINARY SYSTEM

1. a
2. b
3. b
4. d
5. a
6. b
7. c
8. c
9. b
10. b
11. c
12. d
13. a
14. b
15. d
16. a
17. a
18. c
19. b
20. a
21. d
22. e
23. b
24. a
25. c
26. c
27. e
28. b
29. a
30. d
31. e
32. d
33. b
34. c
35. a
36. arteriole
37. Bowman's capsule
38. cortex
39. cystoscope
40. dialysate
41. dialysis
42. dwell time
43. glomerulus
44. medulla
45. nephrolith
46. peritonitis
47. residual urine
48. cloudy
49. uremia
50. urinary incontinence

ANSWERS TO ALTERNATE COMPLETION QUESTIONS

36. nitrogen
37. calyx
38. kidney
39. scanty
40. renal pelvis
41. continuous cyclic peritoneal dialysis
42. end-stage renal disease
43. intravenous pyelogram
44. pH
45. urinary tract infection
46. pus
47. cyst/o, vesic/o
48. -uria
49. ket/o, keton/o
50. meat/o

CHAPTER 16: MALE REPRODUCTIVE SYSTEM

1. a
2. b
3. d
4. c
5. b
6. a
7. d
8. a
9. c
10. b
11. c
12. a
13. d
14. b
15. a
16. b
17. a
18. c
19. a
20. d
21. e
22. c
23. d
24. a
25. b
26. c
27. d
28. e
29. b
30. a
31. e
32. c
33. d
34. a
35. b
36. epididymitis
37. Kaposi's sarcoma
38. prophylactic
39. rectoscope
40. resectoscope
41. residual urine
42. scrotum
43. semen
44. seminiferous tubules
45. spermatozoan, spermatozoon
46. testosterone
47. urethra
48. vas deferens
49. vesicles
50. vasectomy

ANSWERS TO ALTERNATE COMPLETION QUESTIONS

36. male
37. hidden
38. testicle
39. semen
40. balan/o
41. BPH
42. GC
43. IVP
44. STS
45. TURP
46. testicle
47. cry/o
48. prostat/o
49. zo/o
50. sperm

CHAPTER 17: FEMALE REPRODUCTIVE SYSTEM

1. a
2. c
3. b
4. a
5. c
6. a
7. a
8. c
9. a
10. b
11. b
12. a
13. a
14. d
15. b
16. b
17. a
18. c
19. a
20. c
21. d
22. a
23. b
24. e
25. c
26. d
27. b
28. e
29. a
30. c
31. d
32. a
33. e
34. b
35. c
36. menarche
37. menopause
38. menstruation
39. myometrium
40. ovary
41. ovum
42. perineum
43. pregnancy
44. premenstrual syndrome
45. puberty
46. sperm, spermatozoan, spermatozoon
47. uterus
48. vagina
49. vulva
50. tubal ligation

ANSWERS TO ALTERNATE COMPLETION QUESTIONS

36. before (in place)
37. beginning
38. vagina
39. breast
40. men/o
41. metr/o, metri/o
42. ovari/o, oophor/o
43. salping/o
44. -rrhea
45. D&C
46. EMB
47. GYN
48. LMP
49. PID
50. PMS

CHAPTER 18: OBSTETRICS

1. a
2. b
3. a
4. c
5. a
6. b
7. b
8. d
9. a
10. a
11. b
12. c
13. b
14. d
15. a
16. b
17. a
18. c
19. d
20. b
21. d
22. a
23. b
24. e
25. c
26. b
27. e
28. d
29. c
30. a
31. c
32. d
33. e
34. b
35. a
36. edema
37. effacement
38. endometrium
39. episiotomy
40. fetoscope
41. fetus
42. fundus
43. gamete
44. gestation
45. Goodell's sign
46. gravida
47. Hegar's sign
48. labor
49. lactation
50. laparoscopy

ANSWERS TO ALTERNATE COMPLETION QUESTIONS

36. amnion
37. vagina
38. vulva
39. fetus
40. pregnancy
41. milk
42. many
43. -para
44. primi-
45. obstetr/o
46. EDD
47. FHR
48. G
49. last menstrual period
50. normal spontaneous delivery

CHAPTER 19: CHILD HEALTH

1. a
2. d
3. b
4. c
5. a
6. b
7. a
8. c
9. b
10. a
11. c
12. a
13. a
14. c
15. b
16. a
17. b
18. b
19. c
20. b
21. c
22. d
23. a
24. e
25. b
26. a
27. d
28. e
29. b
30. c
31. e
32. a
33. d
34. b
35. c
36. 20
37. growth
38. length
39. lumbar puncture
40. microcephalus
41. neonatology
42. omphalitis
43. tympanic temperature
44. oral temperature
45. pediatrician
46. pediatric nurse practitioner
47. well-child visit
48. crown
49. intussusception
50. patent ductus arteriosus

ANSWERS TO ALTERNATE COMPLETION QUESTIONS

36. embryonic
37. head
38. hidden
39. upon, over
40. water
41. pedi/a
42. omphal/o
43. pyr/o
44. tympan/o, myring/o
45. under
46. SIDS
47. HIB
48. MMR
49. PKU
50. Tb

CHAPTER 20: RADIOLOGY AND DIAGNOSTIC IMAGING

1. b
2. a
3. c
4. b
5. c
6. a
7. c
8. a
9. d
10. b
11. c
12. a
13. c
14. a
15. c
16. a
17. d
18. a
19. b
20. b
21. d
22. c
23. b
24. a
25. e
26. c
27. b
28. a
29. e
30. d
31. d
32. c
33. b
34. e
35. a
36. prone
37. abduction
38. adduction
39. flexion
40. radiation therapy
41. recumbent
42. transducer
43. uptake
44. aortography
45. arthrography
46. brachytherapy
47. bronchography
48. cineradiography
49. irradiation
50. rad

ANSWERS TO ALTERNATE COMPLETION QUESTIONS

36. vessel
37. front
38. joint
39. artery
40. gall, bile
41. sound
42. pertaining to movement
43. luminous
44. back
45. CAT
46. CXR
47. Fx
48. MRI
49. PA
50. PET

CHAPTER 21: ONCOLOGY

1. a
2. c
3. a
4. b
5. d
6. a
7. b
8. b
9. a
10. c
11. a
12. b
13. c
14. a
15. a
16. b
17. c
18. b
19. a
20. d
21. c
22. d
23. e
24. a
25. b
26. d
27. e
28. b
29. a
30. c
31. e
32. c
33. d
34. b
35. a
36. metastasis
37. DNA
38. ionizing radiation
39. mitosis
40. mixed-tissue tumor
41. modality
42. morbidity
43. mutation
44. neoplasm
45. oncogenesis
46. papillary
47. pedunculated
48. relapse
49. remission
50. verrucous

ANSWERS TO ALTERNATE COMPLETION QUESTIONS

36. mets
37. bx
38. PSA
39. TNM
40. RNA
41. cancer
42. chemical
43. tumor
44. flesh
45. hard
46. not, without
47. embryonic state of development
48. change, or exchange
49. tumor
50. nipple

CHAPTER 22: PHARMACOLOGY

1. b
2. a
3. c
4. a
5. c
6. b
7. a
8. c
9. a
10. b
11. b
12. a
13. c
14. a
15. b
16. a
17. d
18. a
19. b
20. a
21. d
22. a
23. e
24. b
25. c
26. d
27. c
28. b
29. e
30. a
31. c
32. d
33. a
34. e
35. b
36. cumulative
37. idiosyncracy
38. potentiation
39. chemotherapy
40. drug
41. pharmacist
42. Hospital Formulary
43. inhalation
44. intradermal
45. intravenous
46. *Physician's Desk Reference*
47. topical
48. buccal
49. transdermal
50. analgesic

ANSWERS TO ALTERNATE COMPLETION QUESTIONS

36. pain
37. cheek
38. drug
39. feeling
40. tongue
41. sleep
42. tongue
43. drug
44. poison
45. a.c.
46. ad. lib.
47. b.i.d.
48. gr.
49. gtt.
50. p.c.

CHAPTER 23: MENTAL HEALTH

1. a
2. c
3. b
4. a
5. b
6. d
7. a
8. c
9. a
10. b
11. c
12. a
13. b
14. b
15. c
16. a
17. c
18. d
19. b
20. b
21. d
22. e
23. a
24. b
25. c
26. c
27. d
28. b
29. a
30. e
31. c
32. d
33. e
34. a
35. b
36. amnesia
37. anxiety
38. apathy
39. behavior therapy
40. compensation
41. compulsions
42. defense mechanisms
43. delirium tremens (DTs)
44. denial
45. family therapy
46. free association
47. intoxication
48. introjection
49. malingering
50. mutism

ANSWERS TO ALTERNATE COMPLETION QUESTION

36. pertaining to a physician or treatment
37. madness
38. mind
39. mind
40. split, divided
41. abnormal fear
42. sleep
43. having a love for, or a strong attraction to
44. emotional state
45. AD
46. DSM
47. DTs
48. ECT
49. I.Q.
50. MMPI

REFERENCES

American Cancer Society. *Cancer Facts and Figures–1998.* American Cancer Society, Inc. Atlanta, GA. 1998.

Austrin, Mariam G. and Harvey R. Austrin. *Learning Medical Terminology: A Worktext.* 8th ed. Mosby Lifeline. St. Louis. 1995.

Beare, Patricia Gauntlett, and Judith L. Myers. *Principles and Practice of Adult Health Nursing.* 2nd ed. Mosby Year Book. St. Louis. 1994.

Benenson, Abram S., Editor. *Control of Communicable Diseases Manual.* 16th ed. American Public Health Association. Washington, D.C. 1995.

Black, Joyce M. and Esther Mattassarin-Jacobs. *Luckmann and Sorensen's Medical-Surgical Nursing: A Psychophysiologic Approach.* 4th ed. W. B. Saunders Company. Philadelphia. 1993.

Bobak, Irene M., and Margaret Duncan Jensen. *Maternity and Gynecologic Care: The Nurse and the Family.* 5th ed. The C.V. Mosby Company. St. Louis. 1993.

Bowers, Arden C. and June M. Thompson. *Clinical Manual of Health Assessment.* 4th ed. The C.V. Mosby Company. St. Louis. 1992.

Brooks, Myrna LaFleur. *Exploring Medical Language: A Student-Directed Approach.* 3rd ed. Mosby Lifeline. St. Louis. 1994.

Bullock, Barbara L. *Pathophysiology: Adaptations and Alterations in Function.* 4th ed. Lippincott. Philadelphia. 1996.

Burgess, Ann Wolbert. *Psychiatric Nursing: Promoting Mental Health.* Appleton & Lange. Stamford. 1997.

Campbell, Linda, Ellen Drake, Sally Crenshaw Pitman, Susan M. Turley. *Medical Transcription: Fundamentals and Practice.* Englewood Cliffs. 1994.

Chabner, Davi-Ellen. *The Language of Medicine.* 5th ed. W. B. Saunders Company. Philadelphia. 1991.

Cohen, Barbara Janson. *Medical Terminology: An Illustrated Guide.* 2nd ed. J. B. Lippincott Company. Philadelphia. 1994.

Collins, C. Edward and Juanita J. Davies. *Modern Medical Language.* West Publishing Company. Minneapolis. 1996.

Comer, Ronald J. *Abnormal Psychology.* 2nd ed. W. H. Freeman & Company. New York. 1995.

Cowling, Cynthia. *Delmar's Radiographic Positioning & Procedures: Advanced Imaging Procedures. Volume II.* Delmar Publishers. Albany. 1998.

Dorland's Medical Dictionary.

Frazier, Margaret Schell, Jeanette A. Dryzymkowski and Sandra J. Doty. *Essentials of Human Diseases and Conditions.* W. B. Saunders Company. Philadelphia. 1996.

Georgiade, Nicholas G., Gregory S. Georgiade, Ronald Riefkohi, William J. Barwick. *Essentials of Plastic, Maxillofacial, and Reconstructive Surgery.* Williams & Wilkins. Baltimore. 1987.

Goodman, Terri. *Core Curriculum for Plastic and Reconstructive Surgical Nursing.* American Society of Plastic and Reconstructive Surgical Nurses, Inc. 1989.

Gorrie, Trula Myers, Emily Slone McKinney, and Sharon Smith Murray. *Foundations of Maternal Newborn Nursing.* 2nd ed. W. B. Saunders Company. Philadelphia. 1994.

Graduate Medical Education Directory. American Medical Association. Chicago, Illinois. 1994-1995.

Greathouse, Joanne S. *Delmar's Radiographic Positioning & Procedures: Basic Positioning and Procedures.* Volume I. Delmar Publishers. Albany. 1998.

Gylys, Barbara A. and Mary Ellen Wedding. *Medical Terminology: A Systems Approach.* 3rd ed. F. A. Davis Company. Philadelphia. 1995.

Ignatavicius, Donna D., M. Linda Workman, and Mary A. Mishler. *Medical Surgical Nursing: A Nursing Process Approach.* 2nd ed. W. B. Saunders Company. Philadelphia. 1995.

Jackson, Deborah Broadwell and Rebecca B. Saunders. *Child Health Nursing, A Comprehensive Approach to the Care of Children and Their Families.* J. B. Lippincott Company. Philadelphia. 1993.

Kinney, Marguerite R., Donna R. Packa, Kathleen G. Andreoli, Douglas P. Zipes. *Comprehensive Cardiac Care,* 7th ed. Mosby Year Book. St. Louis. 1991.

Layman, Dale Pierre. *The Medical Language: A Programmed, Body-Systems Approach.* Delmar Publishers. Albany. 1995.

LeMone, P. and K. M. Burke. *Medical-Surgical Nursing: Critical Thinking in Client Care.* Addison-Wesley. 1996.

Lewis, Sharon Mantik and Idolia Cox Collier. *Medical-Surgical Nursing: Assessment and Managment of Clinical Problems.* 4th ed. New York. 1996.

Memmler, Ruth L., Barbara Janson Cohen, and Dena Lin Wood. *Structure & Function of the Human Body.* 6th ed. Lippincott-Raven Publishers. Philadelphia. 1996.

Mosby's Medical, Nursing, and Allied Health Dictionary, 4th ed. Mosby Year Book, Inc. St. Louis. 1994.

Mosby's Diagnostic and Laboratory Test Reference. 3rd ed. Mosby Year Book, Inc. St. Louis. 1997.

North Carolina Health Careers. North Carolina Area Health Education Centers. Chapel Hill, N.C. 1994.

Pagana, Kathleen Deska and Timothy James Pagana. *Mosby's Diagnostic and Laboratory Test References.* 3rd ed. Mosby Year Book, Inc. 1997.

Phipps, Wilma J., Virginia L. Cassmeyer, Judith K. Sands, Mary Kay Lehman. *Medical-Surgical Nursing: Concepts and Clinical Practice.* 5th ed. Mosby Year Book, Inc. St. Louis. 1995.

Pillitteri, Adele. *Maternal and Child Health Nursing: Care of the Childbearing and Childrearing Family.* 2nd ed. J. B. Lippincott Company. Philadelphia. 1995.

Porth, Carol Mattson. *Pathophysiology: Concepts of Altered Health States.* 4th ed. J. B. Lippincott Company. Philadelphia. 1994.

Price, Sylvia Anderson and Lorraine McCarty Wilson. *Pathophysiology: Clinical Concepts of Disease Processes.* 5th ed. McGraw-Hill Book Company. New York. 1996.

Santrock, John W. *Psychology.* 5th ed. Brown & Benchmark Publishers. Madison, WI. 1997.

Scott, Ann Senisi and Elizabeth Fong. *Body Structures & Functions.* 9th ed. Delmar Publishers. Albany. 1998.

Seidel, Henry M., Jane W. Ball, Joyce E. Dains, G. William Benedict. *Mosby's Guide to Physical Examination.* 3rd ed. Mosby Year Book, Inc. St. Louis. 1995.

Sheehan, Catherine. *Principles and Laboratory Diagnosis: Clinical Immunology.* J. B. Lippincott Company. Philadelphia. 1990.

Sherwen, Laurie N., Mary Ann Scoloveno, and Carol Toussie Weingarten. *Nursing Care of the Childbearing Family.* 2nd ed. Appleton & Lange Publishers. Norwalk, Connecticut. 1995.

Skidmore-Roth, Linda. *Mosby's Nursing Drug Reference.* Mosby Year Book, Inc. St. Louis. 1998.

Sloane, Sheila B. *Medical Abbreviations and Eponyms.* 2nd ed. W. B. Saunders Company. Philadelphia. 1997.

Smeltzer, Suzanne C. and Brenda G. Bare. *Brunner and Suddarth's Textbook of Medical-Surgical Nursing.* 7th ed. J. B. Lippincott Company. Philadelphia. 1992.

Smith, Genevieve Love, Phyllis E. Davis, Jean Tannis Dennerll. *Medical Terminology: A Programmed Text.* 8th ed. Delmar Publishers. New York. 1998.

Spence, Alexander P. and Elliott B. Mason. *Human Anatomy and Physiology.* 4th ed. West Publishing Company. Saint Paul. 1992.

Stanfield, Peggy S. and Y. H. Hui. *Mastering The New Medical Terminology.* 2nd ed. Jones and Bartlett Publishers. Boston. 1995.

Stedman's Medical Dictionary

Taber's Cyclopedic Medical Dictionary. 18th ed. F. A. Davis Company. Philadelphia. 1997.

Thibodeau, Gary A. and Kevin T. Patton. *Anatomy & Physiology.* 3rd ed. Mosby Year Book, Inc. St. Louis. 1996.

Thompson, Eleanor D. *Introduction to Maternity and Pediatric Nursing.* 2nd ed. W. B. Saunders Company. Philadelphia. 1995.

Townsend, Mary C. *Psychiatric Mental Health Nursing: Concepts of Care.* 2nd ed. F. A. Davis Company. Philadelphia. 1993.

Tamparo, Carol and Marcia A. Lewis. *Diseases of the Human Body.* 2nd ed. F. A. Davis Company. Philadelphia. 1995.

White, Lois and Gena Duncan. *Medical-Surgical Nursing: An Integrated Approach.* 1st ed. Delmar Publishers. Albany. 1998.

William , R.W. Basic *Healthcare Terminology.* Mosby Lifeline. St. Louis. 1995.

Wilson, Holly Skodol, and Carol Rne Kneisl. *Psychiatric Nursing.* 5th ed. Addison-Wesley Nursing. Menlo Park, California. 1996.

Practice Software Tutorial

for

Delmar's Comprehensive Medical Terminology

A COMPETENCY-BASED APPROACH

Delmar's Comprehensive Medical Terminology course includes a Windows®-based CD-ROM that contains competency-building exercises and activities. This tutorial should provide enough information to effectively use the *Delmar's Comprehensive Medical Terminology* program. In addition to step-by-step instructions, the tutorial includes several tips, suggestions, and warnings to help you get the most out of the program. The ideas presented here are not exhaustive. We welcome your comments about how you have used the program in your own studies or in the classroom.

The tutorial describes using the various exercises available in *Delmar's Comprehensive Medical Terminology* program. Each chapter has a unique combination of exercises and games. Only the available exercises for a specific chapter will appear in that chapter's window. We recommend that you review the textbook before starting the tutorial, but it is not necessary.

BEFORE GETTING STARTED

Delmar's Comprehensive Medical Terminology program runs under the Microsoft Windows® operating systems. If you have not used the Windows operating system before, you should take a few moments to familiarize yourself with some of its key features. Two important concepts you will need to understand are using the mouse to click a button and using the mouse to select a menu item. Throughout this guide, these two phrases are used to describe the actions you should take.

GETTING STARTED

Before you can use the practice software the first time on a given computer, you need to run the setup program to install key program components to the computer's hard disk. Installing the software is easy to do—just follow the three simple steps printed on the disk label and printed in the back of the textbook. Once the program has been installed, you may launch it from the Windows 95/98 Start menu or from the Windows 3.1 Program Manager, as follows:

- In Windows 95/98: In the Start menu, click **Programs**, then click **Delmar Applications**, and then click **Comprehensive Medical Terminology**.

- In Windows 3.1: In the Windows Program Manager, double click the **Comprehensive Medical Terminology** program icon.

As you proceed through *Delmar's Comprehensive Medical Terminology* program, the last exercises you have studied are automatically saved for you. This allows you to keep track of which chapters you have studied and what exercises within those chapters you have completed. A 3.5" floppy disk is an easy place to have this information stored for you. In fact, the program is designed around having this floppy disk available while the program is running. So, before beginning each study session, just insert the disk in the drive and the program will do the rest. Using the same floppy disk each time streamlines session log-in and ensures accurate results tracking.

Upon launch, the program will display a Welcome window. The Welcome window gives you a brief welcome to the program and asks you to type your name. Because you have inserted a floppy disk in the drive, the Welcome window suggests that you use this disk to store your progress. If this is the disk you want to use to store your progress, type your name, then click **Use Floppy** to continue.

CAUTION: The program CD-ROM must be in the CD drive of the computer in order to listen to the audio pronunciations of the medical terms. *Note:* Your name is printed on the activity reports that you can print on your printer. Since you cannot change the spelling once you have entered your name, double check your typing to be certain your name is correctly spelled before continuing.

CAUTION: Do not remove your floppy disk from the drive until you have exited the program.

The Contents Window

Just as the book has a Table of Contents, so does *Delmar's Comprehensive Medical Terminology* program. The Contents window displays twenty-three buttons that correspond to the chapters of *Delmar's Comprehensive Medical Terminology: A Competency-Based Approach*. To begin work on a particular chapter, click the appropriate button. When you position the mouse cursor over a chapter button, a yellow box with the full title of the chapter appears in the white space near the bottom of the window. Just below the chapter title is a status line. This line tells you whether you have completed any of the exercises in the chapter. At this point, all chapters should state "Not Attempted."

This tutorial will walk you through your first attempt at each exercise and game. Let's begin by exploring the available options in the first chapter, Word Building Rules. Click the **Chapter 1** button to begin this exercise.

The Chapter Window

After selecting Word Building Rules from the Contents window, you will see the Chapter window. This window has a similar appearance for each chapter. So, once you have completed this chapter, you will be ready to study the other chapters in the same manner.

The window is divided into three main areas. The top shows you a picture that represents this section of the textbook as well as the complete title of this chapter. Next, near the middle of the window, there are icons representing the exercises that are available for this chapter. The available selections vary by chapter, and will include a combination of multiple choice, fill-in-the-blank, true false, labeling, matching, or a speed test. In Word Building Rules, the available exercises are multiple choice, fill-in-the-blank, true false, and speed test. Below each of the exercise buttons, you should see a small rectangle with a percentage noted in the center. This percentage shows you how many of the questions you answered correctly in the exercise. When you begin each chapter, these are all set to 0% because you have not yet answered any of the questions.

In the final area near the bottom of the window, the Activities are shown as small icons that represent the three activities. In order across the window, they are pronunciation, board game, and tic-tac-toe. The activities available with each chapter will be bright and bold in color. If you move the cursor over the icon, the name of the game appears below the icon. Inactive activities will have a muted, gray-toned icon, and no name will appear.

Multiple Choice Exercises

Let's try answering some multiple choice exercise questions. Click **Multiple Choice** to begin the exercise. Before starting to answer the questions, take a moment to look at the exercise window. The window appears almost the same for each of the exercises, so you do not have to learn everything anew for each type of exercise. The top of the window reminds you of the chapter and exercise you are currently working on. The right side of the window displays a score sheet. The remainder of the window is used to display the current question.

The score sheet shows the question number and whether you answered correctly on your first or second attempt. A green check indicates that your answer was correct, while a red X shows that you answered incorrectly. The question numbers allow you to jump to any question in the exercise at any time. Click number **5** to see that question. Now, jump back to the first question by clicking **1**. If you want, you can review the full exercise set before answering any question.

Delmar's Comprehensive Medical Terminology program scrambles the questions available to produce one of many possible exercise sets. Even if you see the same question, the correct answer may be in a different position! So, read the question and the answers carefully before responding with your answer.

After reading the first question and the possible choices, make your selection by clicking your answer. You can click anywhere over the text or the corresponding letter button. Immediately, the program tells you whether you are correct or not. Read the information about your answer. If you were incorrect, some clues and hints are given to direct you to the best answer. You then have a second try to pick the answer. If you are correct, you will automatically move to the next question.

TIP: Just type A, B, or C to answer the question.

Try answering all 10 of the questions for this exercise. After you complete the last question, you will have several choices: Study, Restart, Print, and Chapter. Click **Study** to be able to review the answers from this exercise set. Question 1 will be displayed again. To see an explanation of the correct answer, click on any of the answers for that question. Study any of the questions you did not answer correctly by clicking the question number on the score sheet.

After you have finished studying the questions, return to the Chapter window by clicking **Chapter**. The **Chapter** button is found near the top left corner of all the exercise and game windows.

TIP: You can always stop the exercise and return to the Chapter window by clicking **Chapter**.

Fill-in-the-Blank Exercises

From the Chapter window, click **Fill-in-the-Blank** to start the fill-in-the-blank exercise. The exercise looks similar to the multiple choice exercise you just finished. The difference is that you must now type the correct answer in the space provided to complete the given sentence(s). After you type your answer, click **Enter** or press the Enter key on the keyboard. The program grades your answer and tells you whether you were correct or not.

TIP: Remember that spelling is an important part of this exercise, and misspelled words are counted as incorrect.

The score sheet works the same way as it does in the multiple choice exercise. You can go to any question in the exercise by clicking the appropriate question number on the score sheet. Returning to a question that you have already answered shows you the responses you gave as well as the correct answer. Click **Study** to review the explanation of the correct answer.

You do not have to complete all the questions of an exercise before returning to the Chapter window. The program lets you move from one exercise to another at any time. So, you can continue answering all 10 of these fill-in-the-blank questions then return to the Chapter window, or just return to the Chapter window now.

True False Exercise

From the Chapter window, click **True False** to start the true false exercise. The exercise looks similar to the multiple choice exercise. The difference here is that you have only two choices: True or False. If the statement is true, then click **T** or the word **True**. If the statement is false, then click **F** or the word **False**. As with the multiple choice exercise, you can type the letter T or F to indicate your response.

Because there are only two possible answers, you only get one attempt to answer correctly. Read the statements carefully for words like "not," "never," and "always."

The score sheet works the same way as it does in the multiple choice exercise. You can go to any question in the exercise by clicking the appropriate question number on the score sheet. Returning to a question that you have already answered shows you the responses you gave as well as the correct answer. Click **Study** to review the explanation of the correct answer.

You do not have to complete all the questions of an exercise before returning to the Chapter window. The program lets you move from one exercise to another at any time. So, you can continue answering all 10 of these true false questions then return to the Chapter window, or just return to the Chapter window now.

Labeling Exercise

Since Chapter 1 does not have a labeling exercise, we need to change to another chapter. Move back to the Contents window and select **Chapter 4, Whole Body Terminology**. From the Chapter window, click the Labeling button to start the labeling exercise. This exercise is slightly different than the others you have done. The labeling exercise shows a picture with numbered lines pointing to parts of the picture. You need to correctly identify the part by typing its name in the space provided. Like the other exercises, you do not need to identify these parts in numerical order. Simply click on a number to identify a specific part.

You will have two attempts to correctly label the part. After you have completed the labeling exercise, you can either choose to study the correct answers, or to reset the exercise. At any time during the exercise, you can review correct answers or see the correct answer if you gave two incorrect responses by simply clicking on the answer number.

When you are finished, or just ready to return to the Chapter window, click **Chapter**.

The Speed Test

Before selecting the **Speed Test**, be ready to start answering questions immediately! As soon as the first question is displayed, the seconds start ticking by on the clock. The clock is located near the top center of the Speed Test window. Keep one eye on the time and one eye on the question. Answer the multiple choice and fill-in-the-blank questions just as you did for the other exercises. Choose your answers carefully, because you only have one chance to get the correct answer during the test.

Because you probably have not had a chance to complete your study of a chapter at this point, trying to finish the speed test in a reasonable amount of time may be frustrating. As in any exercise, you can stop the test by clicking **Chapter**.

Matching

The window for the matching exercise is slightly different than the other exercise windows. The window is divided into three sections, called panes—two side-by-side columns at the top of the window and a long pane at the bottom. The left hand column lists definitions for important terms and concepts, while the right hand column lists the terms and concepts. To make a match, select a definition from the left column by clicking on it—a highlighted box will appear around the definition to let you know it has been selected. Then click on the matching term in the right column. Correct matches will appear in the matches completed pane at the bottom of the window.

The entire list of choices in either column may not always be visible. To view all the choices, either scroll down the columns or enlarge the panes. To make viewing the columnar lists easier, the panes in the matching window can be resized. To make the matches completed pane larger or smaller, simply click and drag on the pane's top border. When you have completed a matching exercise, the matches completed pane automatically enlarges to allow you to study the correct matches.

RESETTING THE EXERCISES

One more point needs to be discussed before we take a break. The exercises keep track of the last questions you answered and the responses you gave. The speed test even remembers the time on the clock. To start a new exercise set, you need to reset the exercise. The Options menu always contains a Reset command. From the Chapter window, you can reset any one of the exercises. From each Exercise window, you can reset only that exercise.

TIP: Remember that the program scrambles the multiple choice and fill-in-the-blank questions each time you reset. There are so many possible exercise sets that you may never see the same one twice! So, reset the questions as often as you like.

To reset the multiple choice exercise, select **Reset Multiple Choice** from the Options menu. The program asks you if you are certain that you want to reset these questions. Click **Yes**.

TIP: This only resets the multiple choice questions from the current chapter, which is the Introduction chapter in this case.

TAKING A BREAK

Before stepping away from the computer, you should exit *Delmar's Comprehensive Medical Terminology* program. This final step ensures that your progress has been saved on the disk. In the Chapter window, click **Exit**. The Exit button is located near the top right corner of the window.

The program asks you if you are certain that you want to exit. Click **Yes**. Your progress is saved, then the program stops.

Note: Remember to take your disk with you when you leave.

STARTING AGAIN

TIP: Remember to put the floppy disk your work is saved on in the drive before returning to the program.

After putting your floppy disk back in the drive, start *Delmar's Comprehensive Medical Terminology* program by double clicking the icon in the Program Manager. This time the program displays the Contents window directly. You should not see the Welcome window. If you do, then you probably are not using the same disk as before. If you are using a different disk, type your name and click **Use Floppy** to display the Contents window.

ACTIVITIES

Pronunciation, Tic-Tac-Toe and a board game are available for each chapter in the program. The Board Game and Tic-Tac-Toe can also be played as a single player or with two players or teams. You do not have to play the games in any particular order, so you can jump ahead to any of the sections below to read about the game you are interested in.

Pronunciation

Remember: The program CD-ROM must be in the computer's CD drive in order to listen to the pronunciation of terms.

To begin a Pronunciation Activity, click the **Pronunciation** icon. You can also select **Pronunciation** from the Activities menu. Take a moment to become familiar with the Pronunciation Activity window. The top area of the window includes some brief instructions.

Below the instructions, on the left of the screen, is a list of terms. The list shows all of the terms in the chapter for which pronunciation audio is included. The first time you access a list, each term will have a checkmark next to it, which indicates that it is selected.

To the right of the list of terms are two buttons, **Listen** and **Stop.** Click the **Listen** button to listen to the selected terms. After a term is pronounced, there is a pause to allow you to practice pronouncing the term. Using the slider bar located just below the **Listen** and **Stop** buttons, you may adjust the length of the pause to your preference. While listening to terms, clicking the **Stop** button will end the pronunciation set and take you back the top of the list.

If you want to deselect a term so that it will not be included when you listen to the terms, use the mouse to highlight the term and click on it. The checkmark will be removed.

Below the list of terms are **Select All** and **Clear All** buttons. The **Select All** button selects all the terms in the list. **Clear All** deselects all the terms on the list, which will remove all the checkmarks.

Board Game

To start the Board Game, click the **Board Game** icon. It is the second icon from the right, near the bottom of the Chapter window. You can also select Board Game from the Games menu. Your name appears as the first player. Select **Second Player is Computer** to play with the computer's Tutor as the other player. Click **OK** to begin the game.

When playing against the Tutor, you always get to go first. Click **Roll** to begin your turn. After the die roll, you must answer a question correctly to move your piece (the red X). Remember to keep an eye on the timer, too! You only have 25 seconds to respond to the question. If you answer correctly, your piece will move forward the number of spaces shown on the die. If you answer incorrectly, you stay at the same place.

In a moment, Tutor will roll the die and receive a question to answer. While the question is displayed, try to think of the correct answer, too. You cannot respond to Tutor's question directly, but it is good practice to think about the question.

When it is your turn again, click **Roll**. Answer the question. Play repeats until either you or Tutor cross the Finish line. Click **New Game** to start another game.

During your turn, you can return to the Chapter window by clicking **Chapter**. If it is the Tutor's turn, you must wait a moment until it is your turn again before leaving the game.

Tic-Tac-Toe

To start Tic-Tac-Toe, click the **Tic-Tac-Toe** icon found near the bottom right corner of the Chapter window. You can also select **Tic-Tac-Toe** from the Games menu. Your name appears as the first player. Select **Second Player is Computer** to play with the Tutor as the other player. Click **OK** to begin the game.

When playing against the Tutor, you always get to go first. Click any empty square on the board to begin your turn. The center square is a good choice. You must answer a question correctly to place your piece (the red X) in the square. Remember to keep an eye on the timer, too! You only have 25 seconds to respond to the question. If you answer correctly, a red X will be put in the square. If you answer incorrectly, the square is left open.

In a moment, Tutor will pick a square and get a question to answer. While the question is displayed, try to think of the correct answer, too. You cannot respond to Tutor's question directly, but it is good practice to think about the question.

When it is your turn again, choose an empty square. Answer the question. Play repeats until either you or Tutor get three in a row, column, or diagonal. If this does not happen before all the squares are filled, then the player with more pieces on the board wins. Click **New Game** to start another game.

During your turn, you can return to the Chapter window by clicking **Chapter**. If it is the Tutor's turn, you must wait a moment until it is your turn again to leave the game.

NOTES

NOTES

NOTES

NOTES

NOTES

NOTES

NOTES

NOTES